FOOD PASSION PROJECT

A Guide to Repairing Your Relationship
with Food at The American Table

TIFFANY BASSFORD

Published by **◎ FOOD PASSION PROJECT**

To contact the author, visit www.foodpassionproject.com

ISBN 978-1-7322107-0-7
ISBN 978-1-7322107-1-4 (ebook)

Library of Congress Control Number 2018904400

Printed in the United States of America

For my grandmother, who at 19 married into an Italian family and became the best Italian cook I know. She never let your plate be empty, your dishes unwashed, and your clothes not ironed. She taught me that food is, above all, love.

CONTENTS

FOREWORD

"Mom, I think I should have carrots instead."

And so it began. Those words set into motion a lifelong love of food and an analysis of its place in our lives. I was maybe ten when I explained to my mom that I should have carrots for my snack instead of cookies. To this day I can't tell you where that wisdom came from. My mom was shocked at the time and didn't know where the impetus had come for such a bold and mature statement. I somehow knew that carrots were healthier for my body than cookies and that it made sense to eat food that served my body. I was never taught this. I inherently knew it.

To be fair, I never did have much of a sweet tooth. I always said that I'd choose macaroni and cheese over chocolate cake, any day. But carrots? That was a bit of a stretch, even for me. However, from a young age I clearly saw how the food we eat becomes us. I understood that food is what keeps us healthy. I didn't view nutrition in the scientific sense of balancing macros and micros, but in the more basic sense that what we eat directly affects who we become. In my mind, I saw that carrots were natural and mass-produced cookies were processed. My body needed carrots more than processed cookies. Since I had but one body, it was my duty and privilege to care for it. This was so clear even at ten years old.

I grew up in an Italian family where food was, and still is, synonymous with love. There wasn't a family gathering without a spread of entirely too much food. I come from a family where we talk and dream about our next meal while eating our current one. I would have friends join me for such gatherings and they wouldn't understand our obsession with food. I could not understand why they weren't. You mean it's not typical to constantly be thinking of your next meal? However, even coming from a food-loving family, I noticed how family-members (usually the women) would vocalize their anxiety around food and weight.

"I can't even look at the cake or I'll gain weight."

The women would say something to this effect at almost every holiday feast. It never made sense to me. Mind you, young ears are always listening. Why would you make the cake if it's going to cause you so much anxiety? Not to mention, it's a holiday, we don't have cake all the time, so why not have a small piece and enjoy it? You might see this as such simple, childlike logic, but as an adult, I still see food in this way. That cake was made by hand and out of love for a family gathering. The cake does not inherently cause anxiety. We, ourselves, give that power to the cake and to much of the food we eat. Why do we, as eaters, give such negative power to something we require for our existence and ability to flourish? Why do we foster such a poor relationship with something we do three times a day? It always seemed counterintuitive to me. The question remains: why do we do it?

As the family holiday gatherings continued through the years, so did the evolution of family members' relationships with food. I could usually be found within arms-length of the food table. Why? Because I love food. I have a deep, respectful relationship with it. I typically choose to nourish my body with food that I love and is also good for me. However, at holiday gatherings I will destroy a buffet table, expressing giddy excitement over each dish and the variety of flavors available. "I don't understand how you maintain your shape, Tiffany," the women would ask as I typically had some type of cheesy hors d'oeuvre stuffed in my cheek, not minding one bit if I momentarily took on the appearance of a hamster. Did I somehow miss this lesson of being an adult woman? To take your place in adulthood as a woman in America, do you have to subscribe to the notion that you need to deny yourself pleasure in the face of food? Why couldn't you enjoy food but also mind your health and nourish yourself well? Why do we focus so often on a woman's shape? In my mind, nourishment most definitely included both the buffet table and the enjoyment of being with family. I never understood the fallacy that a celebratory meal, or two, would be the ruin of healthy eating habits. I surely don't want to live a life where there isn't room for the gathering of friends and family and the celebratory meal. Again, my logic was this: I make sure I eat well for my body most days, so why can't I become best friends with the buffet table for a day and enjoy extra laughs around it? I also trusted myself to know that I wouldn't continue to eat like that day after day. Celebratory meals are just that: special and a moment to be savored. They're not a door into the abyss of shameful, anxiety-ridden eating. If they currently are that door for you now, please know that they don't need to stay that way.

Trust. That word stayed with me. Do people not trust their body and mind to know how to nourish themselves well? The pursuit of understanding why people eat this way is something that stayed with me throughout my life. Why do people come to the table with guilt, shame, and anxiety? Do people in the rest of the world also face these challenges? What is it about the American food system that encourages unhealthy relationships with food? Why is the state of our public health getting worse and worse as we obsess over the advice of nutritional science more and more? If we were doing something right, then our health would not be failing. I've spent my life trying to answer these questions. While the answers are shades of gray, I refuse to believe that the role of food in our lives was intended to be one of strife. Food can serve as such a source of pleasure, if we just allow it to be.

Diet culture in America has usurped the place where family wisdom on food used to stand. Knowledge about how, what, and in which way to eat food is rarely passed down anymore. There are pockets were this wisdom is maintained and kept alive, but it's slowly fading away and faces continually growing pressures from a broken food system. We've replaced generational knowledge and experience with nutritional studies and "expert" guidance.

My life is a story dedicated to understanding how to repair our broken relationships with food and creating a path to the table that is pleasurable. To this end, I am a food-loving gastronome, a certified international health coach, an analytical observer and researcher of how and why we eat, and a believer in the power of food to change lives. I have lived in Europe twice now: once in Lyon, France as part of my undergraduate degree and once in Bra, Italy to earn my Master of Gastronomy. Both places were so different from my hometown in northern Virginia. In these places, food was love, and it was given a privileged position, held central to the culture and relationships and daily life. I found the intersection of food and life in France to be easy, almost carefree. I walked miles every day in the city, bought groceries more frequently instead of a large haul for the week (influenced by not having a car and only being able to buy what I could carry), and experienced the joy of purchasing my food at farmer's markets. My Sundays consisted of crossing the Rhône and Saône rivers and traveling up to the top of a hill that overlooks the city of Lyon. At the top was Fourvière, a cathedral that remains one of my favorite cathedrals in the world. I'd attend Mass and head back down to the banks of the Saône River where the Sunday farmer's market was abounding. I could wander those stalls forever, soaking in the aroma of the roasting chicken and the potatoes that would lap up their dripping fat (a favorite Sunday purchase for me), examining all of the available cheeses and noticing the excitement of the people crowded around them, taking in the smells of freshly baked bread, and noticing with curiosity the changing fruits and vegetables. A far cry from the sterile aisles of grocery stores in America, Lyon taught me that food is an experience, from start to finish. The purchase of my ingredients, the conversations with the producers, and the celebrations of newly released wines: it was all there to bring pleasure to the eater. And I was free to partake in it!

I promised myself I would maintain these new habits when I returned to the United States, yet I found it increasingly difficult to replicate my French life. I had to rely on my car more heavily as I couldn't walk everywhere I needed to go, and farmer's markets were not as ubiquitous in 2005 as they are now. I returned to the sterile grocery store, never fully releasing the grasp that France had on me. I wanted to understand why I couldn't replicate my French lifestyle and a way of living that served me so well. Upon coming back to the U.S., I saw more clearly the disconnect we have between our food, who produces it, and how much joy food can bring into our lives. Our relationship with food seemed as sterile as the grocery stores in which we shopped. I started researching our food supply to put together the pieces to the question I've sought to answer most of my life: Why do we have such distant relationships with food in America?

After college, I worked in corporate America for ten years and started seeing, and experiencing, more directly how our culture encourages damaged food relationships. The stress, long hours that turned into even longer hours, broken social commitments, sicknesses that came more frequently with increased intensity and duration, and the mental toll of trying to "do it all" eventually landed me at my doctor's office. I was too exhausted to sit up, and my doctor could see my deep fatigue the second he walked into his office. He told me to stay reclined and he'd examine me from that position. I was burnt out and not bringing in enough oxygen into my body. I was ordered to stay home and rest, at least for a few days. Later that day I was resting at home and watching nutrition documentaries (as I tend to do in my free time), and my boss called me in. "Tiffany, I know you're sick," she began, "but we have a client emergency and only you can help." I wasn't just sick. I was exhausted, physically and mentally, but I peeled myself from my couch and, dutifully, into the office I went. I put out the client fire and realized that someone else could have done it in my absence. The corporate definition of emergency was nebulous at best. This is our culture, one that defines emergencies loosely and demands increasing hours and sacrifices of its people. Food oftentimes takes a hit. Too busy to think, we're often too busy to nourish ourselves well, or even to simply make sure we eat. We're making strides to recognize the role of wellness both in life and in the corporate environment, but recognition isn't enough.

I decided to pursue my love of food and nutrition further. Knowing that health was multi-faceted, I attended the Institute for Integrative Nutrition to study over 100 different dietary theories. The study of health, wellness, and the damaged food culture in America encouraged me to start my own health coaching business, Food Passion Project. I combined food knowledge and pleasure into my practice to help those who are trying to do it all and are struggling to find any amount of joy or health at the table. As I coached these women, I remained plagued by how we fail to take care of ourselves in America. There was more to this equation and I turned my gaze to the world to dig deeper. I decided to quit my corporate career, pack up my life (and my cat), and move to Italy to earn my master's degree in gastronomy. There was more to learn about our relationships with food, and I wanted to study in a place that was known for its love of food and the pleasure they take in it. Perhaps there I could find some missing pieces to my puzzle.

Before I left for Italy, I attended an event in support of the health coaching profession on Capitol Hill in Washington, D.C. I told one of the congressmen in attendance that I was leaving for Italy to study healthy food cultures. It was my goal to understand how they come to the table and to then return to the United States to help adapt these lessons to the American context. He nodded in agreement and said, "I sure hope you do. We need it." That statement remains true, perhaps now more than ever. I never forgot this conversation throughout my graduate program. As my studies took me around Italy, back to France, to Spain, Slovenia, Thailand, and Japan, I always traveled with the same questions: How do different cultures come to the table? How can we use these lessons in America to reclaim and repair our relationship with food? I never expected to find a singular answer. Yet, as I shared food at table upon table around the world, I started to see certain habits repeated, and specific characteristics appeared time and time again. There was an understanding of the importance of food—almost a reverence for it. Food pleasure always had a seat at the table.

This is by no means an exhaustive look into how different cultures eat. I even use the qualifying word, *healthy*, a bit hesitantly. My study of healthy food cultures and the research around these areas does not mean that they have uncovered the silver bullet approach to health. In America, we tend to search for the silver bullet answer to health in a pill that will make us lose weight without changes to diet or exercise. Healthy food cultures haven't uncovered anything radically new; in actuality, they've protected the traditions, foods, and customs that have guarded their people well and have been passed down from generation to generation. I observed and researched these characteristics with the goal of making sense of the nutritional confusion that exists in America. I noticed how other cultures come to the table with knowledge of the food they're eating and how it serves them, and they enjoy the presence of those around the table and the food itself. I've included some of these observational anecdotes in this book. I would much prefer to share each of these tables with you because I fear that words cannot adequately capture the feelings I felt around each meal. However, I know that each of these tables changed me, and it's my goal to bring these insights to your table.

It's been said that when you travel, the sights become your insights. These are mine. They have irrevocably shaped the way I view the table and how I approach health and nutrition. As a health coach, they've changed how I coach clients to repair their relationship with food. They've instilled in me a sense of ease with which I approach food. That's why this message is so important to me. I've witnessed the transformation in clients I've coached to help them repair their relationship with food. One client, in particular, came to me with the goal of losing weight. Six months later, she remarked:

"Thank you for changing my life, I have never felt more comfortable in my own skin. There are not enough ways to say thank you. You have changed my life, my relationships, and how I view the world."

I don't know where this book finds you. But it is my hope that it finds you when you need it most. Perhaps you've had a deep sense that your food habits don't serve you. Perhaps you find yourself at the table muttering, "There's got to be a better way." As I traveled the world, I saw that, yes, there is a better way. It's a place at the table with a spread of vibrant, varied real food that begins with gratitude, interweaves pleasure along the way, and ends with connection. I always thought of people back home in America as I experienced the world's tables. If they could just *see* this table, *feel* this human connection, and *taste* this food, they would throw away every diet book. They would understand that the path to health is not paved with deprivation and guilt. In fact, it's the opposite! It's full of delicious, life-giving food, and conviviality. It incorporates who we are as eaters, both the best of us and the worst of us. It's where those two exist in harmony and where the table is not the battlefield. Instead, it's a place where we can learn to make peace with who we are and learn, meal by meal, how to bring our best self to both the table and to life.

Cultivating a healthy relationship with food takes time, unimaginable amounts of trust, and a solid support system behind you. It's a project—a project to discover yourself, bit by bit, bite by bite. The thing about projects is that they're personal; each one changes according to the needs of the work, the team, and the level of experience. That's what is required to make them succeed. As much as our current diet culture would have us think that each journey to health and food freedom is the same, it's not. It's why the table continues to be such a struggle. It's why diets fail us, time and time again. Someone else's food project is not yours, nor should it be. Who you are as an eater is a beautiful part of your story, and the journey to a healthy relationship with food is your project. Your food passion project allows you to unfold the musings of an eater who is trying to find her way and learn who she is. It will be a truthful portrayal of what you feel each step of the way, from angst and sadness to moments of triumphant joy and exhilaration. When I moved to Italy, a friend gave me the sage advice: "Embrace what you don't like with as much gusto as that which you do." Both provide opportunities to playfully explore who we are as people, and now, as eaters. May your project bring you closer to understanding who you are as an eater. The table provides the sacred opportunity, three times a day, to face who we are and who we want to be. It's never just about food. It's always about so much more. It's a conversation with our bodies, the only one with which we were entrusted care. I invite you to join me on this journey to health and to forming a solid relationship with food that is grounded in love, trust, and pleasure.

FOOD PLEASURE MATTERS

I would be a rich woman if I collected money every time someone asked me incredulously, "What do you even mean by a relationship with food? Why do we need to repair it? It all sounds so woo-woo to me." Yet, something that plagues us is typically something we have to face every day. The table provides just that. We talk all too much about diets, new fads, and food labels, but we don't seem to talk enough about who we are as eaters and why we need to forge a strong relationship with food. Our relationship with food is a reflection of our relationship with ourselves and the world around us. It is a relationship that develops and changes throughout our lives. It is a relationship that we must seek to nurture.

In America, we don't seem to have an intuitive sense of what and how to eat. Sure, we have the adage of eating chicken soup when we're sick, but do we know why? Is that knowledge getting passed to future generations? In India, they often eat comforting *kitchari* when sick, a dish consisting of lentils, rice, vegetables, and other ingredients that vary by region. Do we know how to eat to maintain a stasis of health? It has always struck me as odd that we view food as separate from the very vessel in which it will reside. Eating for a sickness comes more naturally because we connect our food to our condition and our hope for feeling better. Eating for recovery from a sickness is also a temporary action. We can commit to it for the few days during which we feel the symptoms of the sickness. We can clearly understand that our body needs good food to help it recover. If we have the capability to connect food to our health, then why do we fail to make this connection after the sickness subsides?

This is where a relationship with food bridges the gap. It's a vital, life-long relationship with ourselves, our food, and why we eat. This relationship can serve as a source of daily stress and strife in your life, or it can serve as a source of gratitude, transformation, and life. It's truly that powerful. A relationship with food is where most diets fail us. Ninety-five percent of diets fail because they're not made for the people who are inclined to attempt to follow their didactic ways. Diets operate as if robots are their target market with their number crunching, tracking of every morsel consumed, and the complete removal of food groups. They don't acknowledge who we are as eaters, the complex beings that we are with all our lightness and darkness alike. We bring our light and our dark to the table with us. It's not left at the door. You might be thinking that this places too strong an emphasis on our food and the table. After all, we aren't entirely what we eat. We're multi-faceted beings with dreams, struggles, deep pains, losses, and passions. We embody so much in this body of ours and all that we embody influences how we come to the table. It influences what we choose to eat, where, how often, and why. Our food becomes us. It becomes our cells. It flows through us. While we embody so much more than just our food, our food becomes a powerful force flowing through all that we think and do. How we eat is how we live. Do we create space for the table or are we too busy, eating in our cars while traveling from meeting to meeting? Do we practice gratitude, or can we not be bothered to think about the source of our food and the work that went into getting it on our tables? Do we honor what our bodies need at the table, or are we too busy meeting other people's expectations to hear what our bodies are asking for?

How we eat is how we live. Think about it. How we come to the table oftentimes mirrors how we show up in life and our cultural environment. Are we thoughtful? Do we make time and space for the things that are important to us? Do we listen to our inner voice when it whispers? Do we respect our voice and our place in this world? Do we honor the one body we're given and how we use it in the world? Do we follow outward diet advice that doesn't sit well with us? Does our culture place emphasis on the importance of mealtimes? Is it culturally acceptable to leave the office and enjoy a meal with friends without the pang of not being "productive?" The list goes on endlessly because how we choose to live is reflected at the table.

One of my clients developed her own ability to eat intuitively and gained more energy to pursue her passions each day; more importantly, she found herself and her voice. How she ate started to impact how she showed up in life. She started facing family issues head on and would defend herself and her life choices to family members, something she previously thought herself incapable of doing. Did the loss of weight suddenly enable her voice? Not at all. In the process of analyzing why she ate and how she was choosing to nourish herself, she was forced to confront a whole host of issues she had buried. Not only had she buried them, she was also using food to numb herself and hide from the gaze of the world. Losing weight made people notice her, remark on her weight, on how she looked. She was an introvert and discovered she was greatly bothered by this attention. By confronting how she was using food to stay more invisible, she was able to confront other places in her life where she wasn't authentically showing up.

After all, how we come to the table is just as important as what's on it. Food, in and of itself, is just food. But we inherently know that there's so much more contained within it and our use of food. As humans, we use food to cope, comfort, and convince. That's not entirely a bad thing as long as we use the opportunity to better understand ourselves. It's how we come to the table and leave the table that is most important. Because it's truly about who we are as humans and what we do in the world with the dreams, passions, and thoughts that are contained in these bodies of ours. The table provides the opportunity to understand ourselves, our actions, and our intentions in a deeply meaningful way. When we learn to respect the power of food and learn to cherish it, we in turn learn to delight in small moments of joy. We send a signal to our brains that we are investing in ourselves, and that we are worthy of care.

Do you think this sounds abstract? Stay with me in this space and we'll work through it together. I'm going to take you to some of the world's tables that I sat around and the food and life lessons I learned from them. We'll discuss the American food system and how that impacts the way we view nutrition, health, and the body. We can't discuss health in a vacuum without diving into our own American culture and how that impacts our opinions, our options, and our access. However, first and foremost, we're going to explore who we are as eaters and how to reclaim our relationship with food, one meal at a time. We're going to do so through the lens of knowledge and pleasure. I've structured this book by focusing on the individual eater first before diving into American nutrition history and how that impacts our relationship with food. This was a deliberate action as I believe that the table provides the opportunity for much self-reflection and insight. Quite frankly, the table is a gift. We need to do this work first before we can look more objectively at the culture in which we live and how it affects us. The work of understanding who we are as eaters combines with the history of American nutrition to build a solid foundation for repairing our relationship with food.

In the current diet culture, we are often taught to be wary of eating with pleasure. Or, perhaps it's our distrust in our own ability to eat intuitively. We fear we'll fall into an ethos of excess when we eat for pleasure. That's where knowledge steps in. By building our knowledge of foods that serve our bodies, we build the ability to feed ourselves and to decipher whether the body is craving greens (it can happen!) or if we really want a cookie and can truly delight in it without any of the negative emotions we sometimes attach to it.

It's important we understand how our diet culture and processed foods alike interact with our bodies because it is impossible to develop an inner sense of how to eat best for our own individual bodies if we don't allow the food to serve us and for our bodies to speak to us. This natural balance is the best way to establish, perhaps for the first time, intuitive eating. Intuitive eating is the space where we respectfully make food decisions with the knowledge of what serves us best at that time, without feelings of guilt or anxiety, while allowing ourselves to experience the pleasure of eating. If you've never experienced intuitive eating, then it might sound too good to be true. We can re-learn how to feed ourselves. I refuse to believe that we were made to count calories and constantly regulate intake and outtake like machines. No. Food is a strong source of human pleasure. We laugh, cry, and share experiences around the table. We can develop intuitive eating to harness the positive power of the table and enjoy one of the pleasures of our human existence. We can learn to understand if we want a cookie, a piece of cake, a spinach salad, or a bowl of soup. Furthermore, we should be able to have the cookie without qualifying it as a splurge, a cheat meal, a fattening food, or a bad food. We should be able to enjoy the salad without labeling it as healthy or a good food. In essence, we place these labels on food; they are not inherently tied to the foods.

This union of eating intuitively with knowledge and pleasure is what I call the *metabolism of passion*. The current nutrition world trains us to be mindful of our caloric intake, to understand the functional role of micronutrients, and to balance our macronutrients all while pointing a judgmental finger if we fall victim to fickle nutrition trends.[1] How we eat is how we live, and this manner of approaching the table makes us anxious, unsure, and guilt-ridden. By reducing food to the sum of its parts (i.e. fats, carbohydrates, proteins, vitamin content, etc.), we have allowed it to become yet another source of anxiety and have removed its power to be a daily source of pleasure. In his book *Nutritionism*, Gyorgy Scrinis provides his thoughts on this manic approach to food: "Recovering or cultivating a sensual approach to food may be an antidote to the obsessive culture of control and the anxieties associated with scientific eating and technologically engineered foods."[2] By approaching food through the medium of enjoyment, we might just find that we can restore our natural relationship with food and resist the toxic notions of our current diet culture. This intersection of pleasure and knowledge is where you cultivate passion at the table. This is your food passion project. It will look different for each of us, but it's one of the most worthwhile projects we can pursue.

Our first experience with food as an infant is one of nourishment and pleasure, two forces which we allow to become oppositional later in life.[3] We are wired to experience food in an enjoyable way, and the food industry knows this. Humans are programmed with incredibly complex bio-computers that beautifully regulate our intake of food and their nutrients to ensure our nutritional needs are balanced. We naturally want to increase our consumption if something is out of balance and is lacking. Alternatively, our body triggers us to decrease our consumption if we overconsume a nutrient. This natural regulation happens behind the scenes, almost without our noticing, but it only works when we consume real foods that our bodies were made to recognize. Processed foods hijack this system by mimicking the flavor of protein through fats and carbohydrates while containing low concentrations of protein. This serves to increase our consumption of fats and carbohydrates as we attempt to eat more protein. The balance of our bio-computer is overthrown as our bodies acknowledge the need for more protein but cannot recognize that the savory taste of processed foods is not providing it. So, we keep eating.[4]

You might be asking, how is pleasure the answer when it is easily overridden? The answer lies at the intersection of knowledge and pleasure. When you make "choices in the light of reason," as described by Carlo Petrini in *Slow Food: The Case for Taste*, then you gain the ability to seek out pleasure in food without falling into an ethos of excess.[5] Passion is the gateway through which we engage food with both our consciousness and our palate. Merriam-Webster defines *passion* as "an intense, driving, or overmastering feeling or conviction."[6] In other words, passion is ambition that is translated into action through the mind, body, and spirit. Merriam-Webster defines pleasure as "a desire, inclination; a source of delight or joy."[7] Pleasure is found in enjoyment, not necessity.[8] Understanding the food system in which we live, paying attention to guttural cues for hunger and satiation, understanding how and why we use food to fill voids, and even making time to shop and cook, are not always enjoyable activities; and in a world of fast and cheap food, it isn't even a necessity. Passion drives these activities from outer influences to the inner gut, a place that is far more resilient to nutrition trends. We then ask our body to metabolize everything we encounter. Our metabolism, the processes that occur within us to maintain life, manages the spectrum of food and emotions we consume and embody.[9] Somewhere between food apathy, the industrial food model, and a reductive focus on nutrients, we realize that another space exists: a space where we maintain life through knowledge and appreciation, both at and away from the table. It is here where the metabolism of calorie-counting gives way to the metabolism of passion. A passionate person perseveres, even when it is difficult and no longer enjoyable. Later, we will explore the broken American food system and how it does not serve to develop intuitive eating. In fact, it fosters distant and broken relationships with food. My hope for the development of food passion is to reignite curiosity in the power of the table and how we come to it.

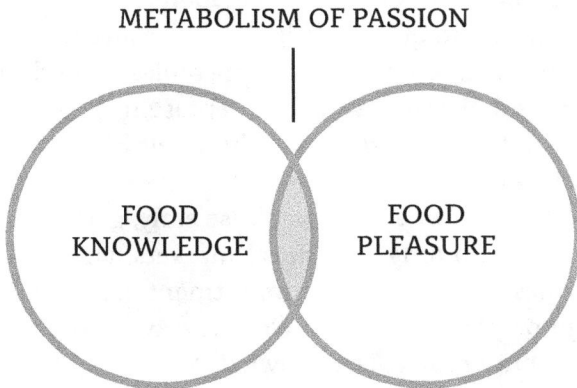

METABOLISM OF PASSION

FOOD KNOWLEDGE   FOOD PLEASURE

Food pleasure matters in that how we come to the table directly impacts how we metabolize what's on it. Thai and Swedish researchers completed a study in the 1960s to understand how preferences impact the body's ability to absorb nutrients. A group of women from both countries were fed a typical Thai meal of rice, vegetables, coconut, and hot chili paste.[10] The Thai group was accustomed to this type of meal and had developed a preference for it. The Swedish women, coming from a different culture, had not, and absorbed 50% less of the iron content, even though the meals were nutritionally identical. The researchers then gave the women a typical Swedish meal of hamburger, mashed potato, and string beans. This time, the Thai women absorbed much less of the iron content as compared to their Swedish counterparts. To take their research even further, they then separated the Thai and Swedish women into four groups. Half of the Thai women received the same Thai meal as before, while the other half received the exact same meal that had been blended together. The same was done for the two groups of Swedish women; half received the same Swedish meal while the other half received a blended version. Both groups who received the blended version of the meal absorbed around 70% less iron than those who received the un-pureed version. The pleasure that the women took in their food, due to taste preferences as well as the form of the meal itself, impacted the nutrition they were able to derive from it. The pleasures of the table and of food actually have a metabolic impact.[11]

This intersection of knowledge and pleasure is also a major theme from my experience with many tables around the world. Knowledge and pleasure were always present. There was also a sense of duty. It was 100 degrees Fahrenheit with a smothering humidity when I was in Thailand, but the families who lived in the rural village where I stayed rose early, gathered the food from their surroundings and local markets, and provided for their families. This level of commitment isn't explained by knowledge or pleasure alone. We know we should cook and provide for our families. The knowledge is there. We also would not typically describe as pleasurable the act of rising before 5 a.m. to fight the impending heat in order to make the first meal of the day. No, pleasure doesn't describe this either. However, the metabolism of passion does. It takes the should and the could and makes it a reality by driving our actions deeper than surface level. The metabolism of passion forces you to examine why you do certain things and the motivations behind your actions. You could even remove the word *Food* before *Knowledge* and *Pleasure* in the model and you'd have a model for understanding life decisions that don't just impact the table. They can stand alone, sure, but their impact on long-lasting behavioral change and a deeper understanding of the self lies in their intersection.

We can no longer combat nutrition confusion with acceptance and trust in a diet culture that encourages damaged eating habits and estranged relationships with food. We are born as intuitive eaters. The metabolism of passion demands that we re-establish our instinctual relationship with food before we lose it completely.[12] It also recognizes food pleasure as a component of healthy living while acknowledging that pleasure does not solve the whole equation. Food pleasure is not necessarily synonymous with excess and unhealthy food choices, nor is enjoying life synonymous with activities that decrease the duration of our lives. I want to live in a world where I can enjoy the cookie and the salad alike, with the knowledge that I'm eating in a way that serves my body. The tables I shared around the world showed me that this is not only possible but is an exceptionally beautiful way of living symbiotically with our environment, our food, and ourselves. By finding peace at the table, we create a passage through which this peace flows more freely into our lives away from the table. When we learn to listen to our hunger cues and to what our body is in need of, we come to listen to ourselves and our inner voice. The table provides the opportunity to tap into this inner voice, a voice we often refer to as our "gut." There's a reason we reference our gut when speaking of our inner intuition. It's there that it lies, if we're only willing to tap into it.

Section I:
WHO WE ARE AS EATERS

We are passion and fury, fire and faith, full of contradictions and everything right. When we breathe in the beauty of our disasters, we allow the good to slowly permeate our being.

How we come to the table is a leading indicator of the state of our relationship with food and, most importantly, to ourselves.

CHAPTER 1

UNDERSTANDING OUR FOOD IDENTITIES

My grandmother's ravioli, a glass of Vino Nobile di Montepulciano, and my grandmother's apple pie.

This would be my chosen last meal. My grandmother married into an Italian-American family at the age of 19 when she married my grandfather. She learned how to cook from my great-grandmother, who came to the U.S. from Calabria with my great-grandfather around the 1920s. My grandmother was the best Italian cook I knew. Even though not Italian herself, her Italian dishes became her children and grandchildren's favorites. At her funeral, I spoke about her food and how it was synonymous with her love: she made food to touch, to smell, to taste. Cooking lessons with my grandmother consisted of my mother in the background quantifying for me exactly what she meant by a pinch, a bit, or add until it feels like a baby's bottom. While I was happy to transcribe the baby's bottom into the recipe I was attempting to capture, I was afraid I'd fall short without more precise measurements. But for her, food was a full sensory experience that requires your taste and presence to do it justice. While some families may inquire about family heirlooms like jewelry, our family could be heard at the funeral musing if she had any of her ravioli in the freezer. When faced with the gut-wrenching task of emptying her apartment, as strange as it might sound, we first raced to her freezer. The ravioli were not there, but the thought of them kept us connected to her.

In my master's program in Italy, a friend of mine would often ask people about their final meal as a way to learn more about them. Try it. Ask your friends and family what their final meal would be. I can just about guarantee that you will learn something about that person through their answers. You almost always will hear a childhood story and learn why a particular dish holds so much meaning. The reason is paradoxically simple and complex.

Food is never just about the food.

Growing up, every Sunday was spaghetti Sunday. I looked forward to it with anticipation each week and never grew tired of it. On the rare occasion my mom would decide to make something else, like a pot roast, we would all protest, "You can't! It's Sunday!" We loved my mom's spaghetti. She would start the sauce in the morning and it would cook all day, weaving its warmth into every available corner of the house. The heavy scent of her sauce still takes me back to cozy Sundays at home, family members moving throughout their day separately, but together. I would sneak, and admittedly still do, into the kitchen to steal a small bowl of the sauce. "Now who took some of the sauce?" my mom would playfully scold the household, even though she always knew the answer. Despite my father working on the car, me and my siblings playing around the house or outside, and my mom moving in and out of the kitchen all day, there was a sense of togetherness in it all. We knew the day would end with family dinner. And spaghetti. Always the spaghetti.

When gluten fear and avoidance became mainstream in the mid-2000s (even though we've known about gluten's identification with celiac since the 1940s) and pasta was frowned upon, I experienced a deeply negative response to it. I was always a nutrition nerd and loved reading about the latest nutritional findings, but this struck a new nerve. The anti-gluten movement was attacking so much more than food for me. It was confronting those spaghetti Sundays at home and the lingering comfort they brought. It placed into question a meal with which I strongly identified, and it was attacking the very foundation of my food memories.

Food is never just about the food.

It's here where nutritional know-how fails us. I'm not advocating a lack of nutritional science; it has served us well over the years. (Scurvy and vitamin C immediately come to mind.) However, when it comes to addressing who we are as eaters and how to incorporate healthy habits into our lives, nutritional science isn't reaching there. Think about your favorite food memory. What comes to mind? What food is it? You might be thinking of a specific dish, or a certain holiday or gathering. Chances are you're also thinking about the people who were seated around the table and the person or people who made the food. I would wager that you're not thinking of the caloric content, the ratio of omega 3s to omega 6s, or what the latest nutritional study said about the healthfulness of the ingredients. Food is about people as much as it's about the food itself. Food is connection, identity, and tradition. Yet, the current state of "eat this but not that" nutritional confusion leaves out the human element of food by myopically focusing on the nutritional components of food. It imagines a world where we make our food selections because of its nutrient properties.

"I'll have the gluten and carb platter with a side of protein and vitamin B12."

That's not how I think of my mom's spaghetti and meatballs. I'd wager that's not how you think of your favorite food as well. As we've established, food memories and our food identity are not tied to nutritional components. It's people who eat, and they eat together, around a table, with food that is meaningful to them. If we remove these vital elements, then we forget why and how we come to the table. If we continue to give nutritional advice that doesn't address why people eat in the first place, then it will continue to not yield sustainable results. The future of American nutrition is rooted in healthy relationships with food, not ever-increasingly contradicting nutritional finds. That future must start first with who we are as eaters. Without recognizing that spaghetti for me is synonymous with love and family, then a basic understanding of who I am as an eater is missing. Thus, the visceral feeling I get when the latest nutritional study tells me that my beloved childhood food is destroying my gut lining. Nutritional knowledge needs to meet me, and you, in that place. This, greatly simplified, is why diets don't work. Diets take away our autonomy as eaters and do not pay respect to the rich history of our relationship with the table.

Often, our beloved childhood foods present a choice of contradictions. It's not just the home-cooked foods that stand in opposition to the ever-growing and changing tide of nutritional knowledge—it's also the processed ones as well. When an oatmeal cream pie carries with it not only familiar flavors, but also the deep comfort of the memories you have of unwrapping it after school, then you face the seemingly impossible decision of letting go of your food memories and food identity with the pie. Simply put, it feels like a betrayal. The food from our childhood brings a level of comfort and continuity. Processed foods, with their mannequin-like components, always offer the same experience. When we reach for them, we subconsciously reach for the memories that accompany them.[1] Continue to eat them, and we defy the advice of nutritional experts; refrain from eating them, and we defy a piece of who we are.

There's a middle ground in this dilemma. Imagine if your mother made a dish that her mother had made. Nutritional knowledge expanded over the years and your mother learned that some of the ingredients contained trans-fats. Yet, she continued to make the dish in the same way to honor her mother. You, in turn, grew up with this dish and are now faced with the same decision: do you make a change to the recipe or pass this along to your children? Would you wish that your mother had changed the ingredients when she learned about their processed attributes? Would your grandmother actually feel honored that this dish had been passed down without change? I believe that we can honor the foods we had as children without passing along damaging ingredients. Let me expand to say that I'm not placing whole food ingredients in this list, like butter. I'm not, by any means, demonizing the role of celebratory foods. We'll cover more on that in chapter 4. We have control over the ingredients we use in our home-cooked foods. Use that power. You can change your mother's (and grandmother's) passed-down casserole to whole food ingredients. Your love and appreciation of this casserole come from the memories you have attached to it. Because you carry those memories as part of your food identity, you can pass along both the memories and the emotions attached to it. Swapping some of the ingredients does not negate that. Allow yourself the freedom to change family dishes out of love and knowledge. As you'll recall, the metabolism of passion works at the intersection of knowledge and pleasure. Use this nutritional knowledge (because not all nutritional findings are controversial) to impact positive change in your life. The food identity you carry with you can endure.

I grew up eating canned vegetables. My preference for vegetables was very much influenced by how much I liked or disliked certain vegetables from the can. I still have a taste for canned asparagus. Even now, I'm immediately ten again, picking up the soggy spears straight from the bowl with my fingers, stealing them from my brother's plate and ridding him of his least favorite vegetable. I now love roasted asparagus with its maintained crispness, but I will never negate the role of its canned counterpart. My parent's food budget didn't allow for a plethora of fresh vegetables; canned vegetables were the most viable option throughout the non-growing months. In the spring and summer, my dad would plant a small backyard garden, and I still remember the tang of the raw mustard greens. I remember shucking corn on the back deck, praying that mine did not contain worms or the cob would find itself tossed by the full power of my young arms. I feel grateful that my mother was adamant about getting vegetables onto the dinner table. Our food identities can honor our past while allowing for changed preferences. We are able to free our food identities to be dynamic components of who we are as eaters. My current food identity is full of fresh vegetables from the farmer's market, delighting in how the seasonal changes bring an abundance of varieties to my table. They change and nudge me into the new season, sometimes reluctantly on my part, but without the colder weather, I don't get my soul-caressing autumn squashes and beloved winter greens; I never would understand the distinctive joy in the salty crunch of roasted and fallen brussels sprouts leaves. I wouldn't fully appreciate the snap of the first asparagus or the creaminess of the spring peas. Eating seasonally enables you to ease through the countless human emotions in a cyclical manner, gently coaxed by the changing crop.

I did not start out this way, but through an investigative mindset, I playfully experienced the world through its myriad tables. An interesting thing happens to your food identity when you travel or live abroad—pieces of it that you didn't even know existed suddenly appear. It first happened when I lived in Lyon, France during my undergraduate degree. The peanut butter cravings hit, and they were strong. I couldn't find a suitable peanut butter in France. The ones I found were too thick and sticky; they didn't have the requisite balance of creaminess and stickiness that I came to know and love. Yet, I continued to buy peanut butter in France. Why? Because it was the flavor of home for me, of Saturday mornings with a thick slice of my grandmother's bread, smothered in peanut butter that warmed from the heat of the toasted bread, dripping through any available holes. Surrounded by an unfamiliar environment with a different language and customs, I was subconsciously craving this comfort and familiarity.

Eleven years later, when I moved from America to Italy, I was older this time and knew the many forms in which acclimation appears. While the food made me feel right at home—spaghetti Sundays were never a problem—I still craved my American comforts. When I came back to the U.S. for the holidays, I made sure to pack light enough to allow for the four pounds of peanut butter that returned to Italy with me. I proudly stacked them in the pantry and rationed one jar per month so that it would last for most of the remainder of my time there. My flat mate in Italy was from Calcutta, India, and oftentimes joked, "You know, Tiff, I'd never know you were American if not for your peanut butter and ketchup obsessions." We carry our food identities with us, sometimes tucked away in our pocket, other times prominently displayed on our pantry shelves—with the lightness of honor and fond memories, or with the heavy burden of pain and shame.

Our food identities are woven throughout our habits and preferences as we determine our tastes and our relationship to food early in life. In fact, most of our taste preferences are established by five years old. What our mothers fed us up to this point determines if we will develop a taste toward processed food, as driven by the early consumption of sweetened baby food, or a taste toward real food. Around the world, there are healthy communities who feed their babies the very same whole foods they themselves consume, setting into motion an inclination toward those foods for life. Members of these communities, dubbed the *Blue Zones* by the National Geographic research team led by Dan Buettner, often live to see 100 years or more.[2] Furthermore, breast milk contains the flavors of the foods consumed by the mother, so through this first touch with the outside world of food, infants are introduced to different flavors. Formula does not provide an ever-changing spectrum of taste, and research has shown that formula-fed babies do not switch as readily to pureed vegetables after being weaned. Breastmilk, as detailed by the research of Menella et al., serves as a "flavor bridge," making easier the transition to adult food.[3]

Infants are pre-wired with taste inclinations to sugar, fat, and salt, and an aversion to bitter and sour. Since processed food is made to appeal to these taste predispositions, it can take multiple exposures to introduce a favorable response to bitter and sour, but research shows that acceptance can ensue with repeated experiences. As familiarity builds, so do preferences. Children imitate what they see and learn from what they experience, from eating socially to food pairings to flavors.[4] It's important that we recognize how a taste for real food (or not) is shaped from a young age. As children, we learn about the food experience through observation, including the place of sensual food pleasure. According to Carlo Petrini, founder of the international Slow Food movement, we are more apt to teach the good/bad dichotomy of food and their corresponding nutritional values than we are to teach the joy of food through the senses. He remarked, "Although the school system is beginning to free itself, however slowly, of the idea that the body is inferior to the mind, there is still a need for a different approach to alimentary education, emphasizing the cognitive capacities arising from sensory experience."[5] From there, Petrini explains, you can awaken their ability to understand what they eat and how they can gather enjoyment from it.

Quite simply, we won't eat what we don't like; and we won't like what we're not exposed to; and if we're not exposed to new flavors then we won't understand the pleasure that can be derived from them. Tastes vary all over the world, from a liking to the iron-rich taste of seaweed in Japan, to a high tolerance and liking for spicy flavors in Thailand. Our taste receptors are the same; the difference lies in our taste preferences and how we register either a favorable or unfavorable response. How we register flavors, as described by food historian Bee Wilson in her book *First Bite: How We Learn to Eat*, travels with us into adulthood.[6] This is not to say that those flavor preferences cannot change, as learning plays a major role in what comes to be identified as food. Our taste preferences hold an amazing capacity for change.

WATER TO SPICE

In my twenties, I dated a guy of Indian descent for many years. I previously did not have a flavor preference for the heavily-spiced food of India. I had never been repeatedly exposed to it. For him, his mother's lamb biriyani held the same place as my mother's spaghetti and meatballs. As I ate his mother's home-cooking over the years, I grew to enjoy it, and then crave those flavor profiles, and then like it so much as to cook it myself. One thing stood in my way: the heat. I loved the food his mother made, and I often told her I wanted to eat it just the way she made it, but I knew she cut down on the chilies when I was at the dinner table. Still, I would gulp down my water, as inconspicuously as I could muster (i.e. not inconspicuously at all), much faster than anyone else at the dinner table.

Tired of embarrassing myself by my lack of heat tolerance at the table, I took this as a challenge. I set out to increase my tolerance of heat, bit by bit. I would seek out spicy food of increasing degrees and sweat and gulp my way through it. I was determined to enjoy the dishes the way they were prepared. For a year and a half, I took to this challenge. Around the one-year mark, I started to crave spicy food. In my 25 years of life at that point, I had never craved spicy food, but here I was, thinking about my next meal—a common occurrence—and I was craving spice. Victory! I had successfully changed my flavor preferences.

I now understand what was happening to my body at that time. Because of the capsaicin in chilies, our bodies interpret the sensation we experience as warmth. Our brains compensate by releasing endorphins to help relieve the pain and soothe us through the experience. Endorphins are addictive, which explains why I started to crave spicier and spicier foods as I proceeded through my experiment.

With my newfound love of heat, I could unabashedly explore a whole new world of flavor experiences. When my graduate program took me to Thailand in my thirties, I fondly remembered my pursuit of spice and was ever-thankful as I consumed bowl upon bowl of chili-laced curries.

Our food memories can define our identities as eaters, but they are merely chapters in our books, not the entire book. I hope this chapter has established that our food identities provide valuable insights, but they are also malleable. Food carries with it a plethora of memories and emotions and has the ability to shape our identities as eaters. Understanding your food identity provides valuable insight into how you relate to food, which foods are important to you, and why you continually reach for certain foods. Understanding your food identity is the first step in reclaiming your relationship with food. Use the provided activities at the end of this chapter to begin to understand your own food identity. Approach every activity from a place of curiosity and amusement. Do not pass judgment on yourself or your answers. Take this opportunity to learn about your food identity and how it impacts your relationship with food. The journey to cultivating a healthy relationship with food begins with the knowledge of all that you carry to and from the table. By understanding how and why you come to the table, you build confidence in your ability to approach it with knowledge. You release the table of the hold it previously held over you.

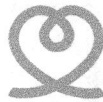

SUGGESTED PROJECT: WHAT IS YOUR FOOD IDENTITY?

Ask friends and family about their chosen final meal. Share what yours would be and why. Think about how your food memories shape your current relationship with the table.

- What foods did you eat growing up?

- What foods do you eat now?

- What are the foods you turn to for comfort?

- What foods do you make that are passed-down family recipes?

- How do these insights impact your food identity?

- What part of that identity serves you and what part no longer does?

CHAPTER 2

ON KALE AND QUINOA

I want you to be everything that's you, deep at the center of your being.

CONFUCIUS

We've been bombarded by a plethora of information on what to eat, when to eat, when not to eat, what we were once told to eat but are now being advised to no longer eat. It's maddening. If nutritional know-how was the missing link, then we'd just eat our veggies, moderate our meat, and carry on with our lives. According to the 2017 OECD Obesity Update report, obesity on a global scale is the highest in the United States.[1] Paradoxically, the U.S. seems to focus more on health than other countries in which I've lived or visited. We're the land of kale, quinoa, and green smoothies as much as we're the country of abundance, large portions, and excess. We operate in extremes in an attempt to find the balance that eludes us. In America, we try to force consumer culture and mindset onto health. If we only do more, try harder, buy more health products—where does it end? Healthy living is not all about nutritional knowledge, but how and why we're eating. Notice there is a deliberate omission of the word *what*. We already focus too much on this word: what we want to look like, what foods we're eating, what foods we're not eating. Lack of information is not why we're facing increasing rates of obesity and food-related illnesses.

Our frenzied approach to nutrition matches our frenzied approach to dieting and to how we live our lives. Life is disproportionately fast in America and yet, we're advised to do more for our health. What if the answer lies in doing less? Does it sound illogical to you? Stay with me. Doing more does not change the negative behaviors we've spent years building into our lives. We need to do less of what does not serve us: less of the negative self-talk, less of the frenzied eating on the way to a meeting we don't even want to attend, less of the exercise out of punishment for what we ate while rushing to that meeting. Enough.

I always tell my clients from the start: I can talk to you about the benefits of kale and quinoa until I'm blue in the face, but if we don't discuss the fact that you're an emotional eater and you're struggling with marital challenges that are triggering your nighttime eating, then we won't get anywhere meaningful. Sure, you might incorporate a bit more kale and quinoa into your diet, for now, but you will not understand who you are as an eater and why you're reaching for late-night food to soothe wounds that won't be healed through the fork.

Do less. By doing less, you make space to fill it with good. We cannot create healthy habits without first creating the space in which to house them.

Once we create that space, we need to be mindful of how we fill it. All too often, we invite restriction and willpower to gather in that space. We treat willpower like the sole thread connecting us from where we are to where we want to be because we can't conceive how that chasm can be filled by gratitude, appreciation, and pleasure. Willpower is a finite muscle and, like any other muscle, it will eventually fatigue. Furthermore, where we want to be is an expression of *what* we want to be. When it comes to food, *what* we typically want is weight loss and an embodiment of the culturally accepted thin frame. We then use willpower and restriction in feeble attempts to reach something we think we want.

Fad diets lie in the *what*. They market and speak to the *what*. You know this because you see it plastered everywhere: the toned abs, minimal hips, small frame, and the smiling faces. They speak to the cultural ideal that being thin means being happy and they dangle it in front of you disguised as health. True healthy relationships with food lie deeper than that; they exist in your *why*, not your *what*. Why do you want a healthy relationship with food? Is it because it will enable you to have the energy you desire to be present with your children while still pursuing your own passions? That's your *why*. What you do to get there can look different on any given day but knowing and tapping into your *why* is what keeps you close to your center. What you do to attain a healthy relationship with food might look like grilled vegetables and roasted chicken one day, pizza another day; it might look like a 30-minute exercise that you enjoy, or it might look like a nap. It lies in our ability to tap into what our body needs at any given time. This builds confidence in our decision-making abilities, trusting that we are shaping our lives around what is most important for us.[2]

I often ask my clients 'Why?' seven times, or as many times as it takes, to peel back the layers and understand their true motivation.

Client:	I want to lose weight.
Me:	Why?
Client:	I've been overweight all my life and I'd like to be thin.
Me:	Why?
Client:	I have a hard time fitting in and think it would be easier if I were thinner.
Me:	Why?
Client:	People seem to relate to thin people differently than me.
Me:	Why?
Client:	I can be a bit awkward in groups. I've struggled with social anxiety since I was young and never truly overcame it. I've just learned to mask it with food. I'd like to be able to be confident in social interactions.

Now we have something to work with. Kale and quinoa could never have made a dent in this. It's of no fault of their own. They just can't reach where this wound is. At least, not yet, because hunger is the absence of something. We just need to do the work to figure out for what we are actually hungry.

A client came to me to lose weight. (This is a common theme among my clients as a result of diet culture and the challenging American food system in which we live.) She voiced that she wanted to finally feel comfortable in her own skin. We oftentimes think about comfort in our own skin from external standards of size and beauty. Only then can we be comfortable in our frame, we think. However, that which plagued you before does not disappear with a smaller frame. If so, models would be reported as the happiest people on earth. (They're not.) My client didn't know what was lying underneath her request to feel comfortable in her own skin, but it was a plea for permission to acquiesce into her authentic self. Starting small, we built her confidence in herself and in her ability to make decisions that serve her. Reluctant acceptance of new habits gives way to a deeper permission to introspect, and introspection leads to curiosity in the self.

At the end of our program, this client remarked how she came to me to lose weight but that we didn't talk about food for long. We talked about everything surrounding the food. She had no idea that her unhealthy relationship with food pointed directly to spaces within herself that required healing. The most important weight that she lost was the weight of carrying around a negative self-image. Most of our work is in our inner mind, not the table. The table simply allows us to access this work multiple times a day.

Food triggers take many shapes and forms. They're as unique as we are as eaters. As we discover who we are as eaters, we begin to understand how we interact with food. Do you find yourself reaching subconsciously for chocolate when you're upset? Once you understand how your food identity impacts your relationship with food, you enable yourself to move the subconscious action to the conscious. This allows you to understand yourself more fully the next time you find yourself reaching for chocolate. *Pause. I'm reaching for chocolate. I'm upset and hurt today. What is my body asking for?* There's nothing inherently wrong with enjoying a soothing piece of chocolate when you're upset. Ask any nutrition nerd and we'll be the first to tell you that we each have a lovingly stocked part of our pantry with our favorite high-quality chocolates. The point is to tenderly know and understand your *why*, not inflict more turmoil on your body by restricting the chocolate. This can play out in multiple ways:

Pause. I'm reaching for chocolate. I'm upset and hurt today. What is it my body is actually asking for? I'm looking to feel loved and appreciated. While I recognize that the chocolate cannot provide that, I do truly desire to enjoy a piece of chocolate in this trying moment. I will enjoy the chocolate without guilt, shame, or anxiety.

-Or-

Pause. I'm reaching for chocolate. I'm upset and hurt today. What is it my body is actually asking for? I'm looking to feel loved and appreciated. I'm not even hungry and do not want the chocolate. I'm going to take a long bath to allow myself to breathe. While I feel that I'm lacking outward expression of love and appreciation, I will start with the inner work of loving and appreciating myself.

These are two examples of how understanding your food triggers enables you to better understand yourself. Neither of these responses is better than the other. Each one is a perfectly loving response. They also allow for the full expression of what it means to be human and to navigate the whole realm of emotions that we bring to the table. A healthy—and human— relationship with food is grounded in flow and pragmatism: too strict and you feel the pressure of perfection; too loose and you lose yourself.

More knowledge doesn't address our need to be human in our expression with food. It does not single-handedly address our food identity, how we grew up, the tastes we grew to prefer, or how the diet industry fuels our fears. We can take the information we learn about ourselves and use that, little by little, to understand more about how and why we come to the table. We'll speak about what healthy food cultures have on the table a little later, but we need to first understand and love the person who will be sitting at the table.

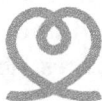

SUGGESTED PROJECT: FIND YOUR WHY AND EXAMINE FOOD TRIGGERS

- Ask yourself "Why" as many times as it takes to figure out your true motivation behind desiring a healthy relationship with food. This can take many iterations to uncover your why. That's OK. Sit with your answers and come back to them later. Like an onion, there are often more layers to peel.

- What foods do you reach for when you're upset / sad / happy / struggling / depressed?

- How can you reframe your food triggers into opportunities to provide the nourishment your body is asking for?

- How can your food triggers serve you by allowing for a deeper understanding of your food identity?

CHAPTER 3

THERE'S A HOLE IN MY BUCKET

"There are only two types of people in the world: those who try to stuff their inner emptiness, and those very rare precious beings who try to see the inner emptiness. Those who try to stuff it remain empty, frustrated. They go on collecting garbage, their whole life is futile and fruitless. Only the other kind, the very precious people who try to look into their inner emptiness without any desire to stuff it, become meditators."

OSHO[1]

I remember gleefully singing a song as a child about a man who needed to fetch water but found that there was a hole in his bucket. His wife told him to fix it with straw, but the man needed to cut the straw, which required an ax that needed sharpening, and the stone to sharpen the ax needed to be wet, which required water. The song concluded comically as the man arrived back to the main point: he could not gather water because of the hole in his bucket.[2] When I sang this as a child, I would giggle over the sheer lunacy of it all. When I think of it now, I see how we oftentimes have holes—whether it's depression, a broken marriage, or wounds we carry with us from childhood—that we try to fill with food, but the food never quite plugs that hole. The temporary relief of eating soon subsides to guilt, shame, and anxiety. It serves to widen the hole we're trying to fill. In an attempt to fill the ever-widening hole, we eat again and again. The binge/

restrict spectrum exists for a reason. It biologically prevents us from ever settling into one end of the spectrum because the extremes are not where we belong. We need to strive to have that pendulum settle near the middle. I don't say *in the middle* because it implies food perfection, and that does not exist, nor should it. By keeping the pendulum near the middle, it allows it to swing to the indulgence side of the spectrum for celebratory meals. It also allows it to swing to the restrictive side of the spectrum when we're ill or simply not as hungry. Imagine a rubber band attaching *binge* on one side to *restrict* on the other, with *intuitive eating* in the middle. When we put more and more pressure on the band as we move closer and closer to restriction, the band will eventually have too much pressure and catapult us to the binge side without stopping in the middle. How could it? There was simply too much pressure.

In writing about the role of taste in society, Jean Anthelme Brillat-Savarin notably provided us the quote, "Tell me what you eat and I shall tell you what you are."[3] This was not intended to indicate that you literally become what you eat, but how and what we eat is an expression of who we are. Food communicates how we feel about ourselves. When we overly restrict food, what messages are contained within it? Are you trying to communicate that you can control your life and that you embody the cultural ideals of thinness?[4] When you binge, what messages are contained therein? These messages contain the answer to what we truly need to fix the hole(s) in our bucket. That's the work we need to be doing in order to approach the table with confidence. The majority of the work to reclaim our relationship with food usually occurs away from the table. That's why diets fail; they start with the table. However, food is oftentimes not the hole in our bucket; it's the straw with which we're trying to plug it.

I typically coach clients for a minimum of six months and up to several years. As their lives change and they encounter new challenges, it serves them to have support and guidance along the way. I typically see clients self-sabotage their efforts around the four-month mark. Why? They're still establishing new habits, and until we get to the bottom of what their "hole" is, old habits will creep back in. I had a client who was working hard to establish a healthy relationship with food. She was a teacher and was also earning her master's degree at the same time. We first worked to overcome her sugar addiction to allow her to taste the beautiful, natural sweetness of a strawberry. By tackling this first, we were able to make peace with a source of her daily struggle and a catalyst for food choices that no longer serve her. It was also robbing her of her natural stores of energy, and it's difficult to make any changes when you simply don't have the energy. She began to increase her recipe repertoire and find and make recipes that were delicious and doable in her and her husband's hectic schedules. She was feeling more confident in the kitchen and in her ability to feed and invest in herself. She took pride in achieving a perfect sear on her food, something she told me she would never have previously imagined. Her "hole" was slowly being filled as she established new habits that served her, and the confidence that was derived from them. The healing was aided by her newfound skills, but, as we've discussed, lifetime healthy habits are built when we tackle the *why* behind it all. Oftentimes, this work brings new things to light.

As she was arriving at a natural weight for her body, people would comment on her appearance. "Oh, you look great!" "Wow, what are you doing to lose weight?" These seemingly innocuous statements had an unconscious effect on her. She experienced a month of struggling in a way she hadn't experienced since we first started working together. In areas where she previously felt excitement and motivation, she now felt burdened and troubled. In one particular session, we spoke about the root of these feelings. We didn't talk about strategies to incorporate healthy food into her days. That would put the focus on the *what*, we needed to focus on her *why*. She already had the knowledge of what to eat. We had to uncover why she was self-sabotaging her efforts.

As it turned out, the answer was buried more deeply than either of us expected. As people remarked on her appearance, she felt visible as she moved throughout her days. A lifelong introvert, she felt uncomfortable with this level of attention. As we talked, she realized that she never felt comfortable with her introversion. In an extroverted world, she always felt apologetic, less than in some way, because of her introversion. This newfound visibility made her aware of her discomfort with being center of attention. She continued digging. In fact, at a larger body size, people did not comment on her appearance. She felt like she could move more invisibly throughout her days. All of a sudden, people found her appearance something they could comment on. Well-intentioned, they complimented her visible external work. What they couldn't have known is that their comments were also spurring a ton of inner turmoil.

My client took this insight and began to investigate why she was trying to hide behind her weight. Her self-sabotage now made sense to her. She could identify what the "hole" was and started the work of filling it more permanently, without the use of food. She began the work of honoring who she was and her natural inclinations. Her road to a repaired relationship with food was paved by an acceptance and appreciation of her intro-version, and a slow but steady build in her ability to own who she is and her voice. She found herself stating her needs with a surety of which she had previously thought herself incapable. She found and owned her voice, and that will always be more important than the number on the scale. With this discovery, she learned more about who she is as an eater and as a person. In other words, she uncovered her *why*. Why did she want to repair her relationship with food? Because she wanted to love herself enough to know that she was worthy of nourishment, worthy of love, and worthy enough to own her voice.

We don't come to the table with the same motivations and stories. Food would have never filled this "hole." Try as we might to avoid it, we have to do the work of an investigator. Our path might be just as convoluted as the song lyrics at the beginning of this chapter. Unlike the bucket, the journey to uncover your "holes" and their permanent fixes is the journey to learn more about who we are. It's a meaningful investigation that serves you for years to come.

Our cravings in life provide indications for what we are seeking and our desires. Cravings at the table can also provide needed inputs. Our culture teaches us to fight our cravings and to not give in. We are trained to judge cravings as weakness and to see our ability to resist directly correlated to our strength of character. Can we establish once and for all that this is absolute nonsense? Our cravings are beautiful beacons that enable clear insights into what our body is asking for. Like any language, it is conveying information. It just happens to be a language we were not taught. In fact, we were taught this language incorrectly. Our body might be craving the chocolate cake. We interpret this incorrectly as a weakness that we are plagued with thinking about cake again. We interpret this as a moral failure.

The error is not in the thought itself but in our interpretation. It reminds me of when I was traveling and trying to stumble my way through multiple foreign languages. Once I was gaining confidence in my Italian abilities, I would still find myself answering emphatically, "Si!", when someone was asking about my preference for the time of the dinner party.

An Italian friend, in Italian: "Tiffany, what do you think for dinner tonight? Should we do 7 or 8 tonight?"
Me: "Si!"

The error was not in their questioning but in my ability to interpret. I was able to understand that she was asking me about dinner that evening. I took those few words and deciphered them as, 'Do you want to have dinner tonight?' While less cheek-flush inducing, our inability to interpret bodily cravings is equally comical. You are not inept because of your inability to read your own body any more than I was to blame for misunderstanding a question in a language I was trying to learn. I simply had not yet learned the words, but each encounter was an opportunity to improve, to learn, and to interpret more fluently. The same with our cravings. We need to learn to become more fluent in the language of our bodies.

I had a client who was a mindless eater. She would come home from work and immediately grab something to eat, whether or not she was hungry. We worked together to establish a line of communication between her gut and her actions. If she came home and felt the strong inclination to grab a brownie from last night's bounty, she learned to pause and think about what her body was actually demanding from her. On one occasion, she realized that she had a particularly challenging day and was tired and worn down from the day's activities. She left the kitchen and took a long shower, detaching herself from the day and pampering her body with self-care. When she came back downstairs, she forgot that she had wanted the brownie an hour earlier. Once more in the kitchen, she thought about what her body really needed, and she no longer felt the craving for the brownie. She didn't resist out of restriction or deprivation. She simply gave her body what it was truly asking for.

The bottom line is this: I want you to want to feed your body nourishment out of love. Again, I want *you to want* to feed your body nourishment out of love. It doesn't mean anything if I want you to, or if the newest diet wants you to, because those are always coming from an external place and a sense of duty. Health can't develop from a place of dutiful fulfillment. Instead, it blossoms in an environment of careful fostering. Let's face it, things will always arise, and challenges will always present themselves. These are all opportunities to examine our *why* and what we want out of life. They are all beacons to hone in on exactly what matters to us. Healthy lifestyles are not always the easy or most desirable choice. When we make decisions from a place of knowledge and pleasure, the metabolism of passion kicks in and we persevere, even when we don't want to. When we truly honor ourselves, we honor our challenges. We honor our muck. We thank it for allowing us to do the work of digging deep and figuring out what we're about. That's where the deep healing occurs.

We look at health as an event that happens at some preordained time in the future. Yet, we acknowledge that we need to feed and bathe our children regularly, and we need to water the plants consistently. Why do we not carry that language over to the feeding and caring of ourselves? We oftentimes think of approaching health as this restrictive event for which we need to prepare our mind. The only preparation you need to do is to speak loving words to yourself; the rest will follow. When you deem something worthy of care, you tend to it. The same goes for how we approach the table.

With each food encounter, you gain an opportunity to speak the language of your body, to understand it better, and to interpret its language more fluently. What an amazing opportunity! The table provides a meeting space for us to better understand ourselves. Come to the table, each day, with a willing heart to discover what your body is asking you to provide. Many times, you might just find that it's asking for something that can't be provided by the table. Nourishment happens away from the table as much as it occurs at the table. Nourish. Listen. Act.

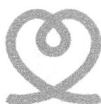

SUGGESTED PROJECT: LEARN THE
LANGUAGE OF YOUR BODY

For the next week, approach your food decisions with amusement and curiosity. No judgment. No shame. No guilt. Just amusement and curiosity.

For example, did you come home and automatically reach for a leftover cookie? Interesting. Why did I reach for the cookie? Was I hungry? Was I bored? Was I actually looking for comfort? Could a warm bath or an engaging conversation with my partner have fulfilled what I actually need? Lead with amusement and curiosity, always. Remember, the point is not to talk yourself out of the cookie, but to bring the conscious to the subconscious.

CHAPTER 4

CAN WE TALK ABOUT THE CHOCOLATE CAKE?

When autumn darkness falls, what we will remember are the small acts of kindness: a cake, a hug, an invitation to talk, and every single rose. These are all expressions of a national coming together and caring about its people.

JENS STOLTENBERG[1]

I was eating a *salade Lyonnaise* outside a café in Lyon on a warm July night. I didn't want the fact that I was traveling alone to deter me from visiting my favorite street in the city, rife with little cafes and restaurants wedged next to one another for the entire length of the avenue. I opted for the *prix fixe* menu so that I could enjoy a few of the dishes that garnered Lyon the title of gastronomic capital of the world. A place that can make a crave-worthy salad is a place in which I want to be eating. There I was, savoring each fatty and meaty piece of the *lardons* laced with just enough of the warm vinaigrette, taking in the scenery, the people who walked by, and the plate in front of me. I have had many moments in my life as an eater that have made me stop and take in the experience. This is what food pleasure is about. These moments make me feel so far away from my home country where we place an emphasis on calories and balancing our intake and outtake. This moment captured for me the power of the table and how we come to it. I took no guilt into this meal and no shame away from it. I was present and dedicated to the experience, even with my discomfort of dining alone. With each bite, I was transported further and further to a place where food enjoyment was permitted, encouraged even. There was no gluttony and no self-reproach, only full permission to be present and drink in the experience.

This got me thinking: there's something to this. Actually, there is a lot to this. We're not oftentimes (or ever) dining at a café in France, but the lessons of food pleasure remain, and France is a place that is notoriously comfortable with taking pleasure in food. For the French, good food is a way of life. They see a clear connection between a good life and good food. If it's possible to experience such pleasure at the table, then how can we harness that energy in America? How can we rid ourselves of the fear that enjoying our food will encourage us to eat too often, or to overeat when we do? We seem to fall into a self-imposed balancing act, where the more we take pleasure in our food, the higher our risk for excess. Why do we treat food pleasure and health as mutually exclusive entities? They're not, nor should they be. We won't be in equilibrium if we stop enjoying our food a bit more. As I brought this question with me to each class, to each client, and to each table around the world, I noticed two trends emerge.

1.   Healthy food cultures pair food knowledge with food pleasure.

2.   Healthy food cultures have real food on the table.

Let's examine point one first. When I was living in Italy, my Italian friends would ask me why we fear pasta so much in America. They would emphasis that pasta is life for them. It's the ravioli of their *nonna*, the spaghetti of their *mamma*. They would explain that they don't have pasta every day, sometimes not even a few times a week. When they do eat pasta they typically have a smaller portion and eat something else with it. There was an ease with which they approached the topic of pasta. With a simple shrug, they conveyed: eat good pasta, enjoy it, and don't eat too much all the time. How realistic an approach. They give themselves permission to eat good food while understanding that one good plate of pasta does not mean it needs to be repeated daily.

Dan Buettner's National Geographic research team found that the world's healthiest food cultures understand the role and importance of the celebratory meal.[2] A celebratory meal might be a Sunday or holiday meal, and it is typically categorized by more food, and richer food at that. You don't hear people remark that they shouldn't eat such and such. They understand the role of the special meal and its place in their life. Sometimes we look at those meals as the final straw to an already poor diet, the meal that will destroy the last remaining of our "healthy" intentions. Airplanes course correct from takeoff to landing. As different factors constantly throw them off course, pilots make small adjustments throughout the flight to land in their final destination. They can't fly without the air, but the wind also changes their trajectory. Airplanes need to make adjustments to adapt to the very thing they require in order to soar. We are no different with our food.

Every time I hear someone remark that they shouldn't eat something, I'm brought back to the chocolate cake from my youth. We require chocolate as much as asparagus. OK, maybe not in a biological sense, but in the place where a grilled cheese and tomato soup envelops your soul and wraps it in deep satisfaction. It's the meal that you eat in that rare moment where your biological functions meet your soul. Every so often we hit that place and we know when we do. We don't forget those chance meetings. The purpose of eating with knowledge and pleasure is to tap into that place where we understand what our body needs biologically and what is required to sooth our soul. It's about changing our approach from gritting our teeth to surrendering more. The celebratory meal does not need to set us off course and make us abandon our path. It's less about what we do between Christmas and New Years and more about what we do between New Years and Christmas. Don't sweat the celebratory meal. They, too, serve their purpose. They provide punctuation to our years, moments to bring people together around a table filled with food that we love. And if that table holds homemade chocolate cake, have some. Please.

Healthy food cultures recognize when the celebration ends, and the role of food graciously shifts to the day-to-day fare they typically consume. They don't switch out of self-punishment for the indulgences they had, nor do they change their food from a place of reluctant obligation. They simply acknowledge that there is a time and place for everything, and everything has its purpose.

Turning to point two, healthy cultures have real food on the table. This point is the one that struck out to me most through my travels and experiences living abroad. It's deceptively simple. Pasta in Italy is made with high quality grains and laced with freshly made sauces. Curries in Thailand are made with seasonal vegetables that radiate life in their flavor. Fast food in Japan is made with regional ingredients and a proper *dashi*, or broth. It's all food that is minimally processed and, for the most part, seasonal. It's not made in a facility far away and delivered in ready-to-serve microwavable containers, passed off as homemade in some back kitchen. The food was simply less adulterated, and it had flavor. Spinach in Italy is some prehistoric cross between Jurassic kale and the spinach that we know. (OK, it's not, but it has more flavor in a single leaf than I've ever experienced before.) It has a bite and a flavor that announces itself as spinach. It's not meek or timid in its identity as spinach. When I want spinach, I want that. It didn't stop at the spinach: the tomatoes were sweeter and soul-quenching. They enveloped everything a tomato should be. It's no surprise we're not satiated by our food in America. Flavor in food is the expression of its nutrient content, and a water-logged tomato isn't doing much for me. Or you. We are creatures that crave flavor. It's our biological pursuit of nutrition in summer-ripe tomato clothing. The more you are able to enjoy the flavors of real food, the less you reach for the food industry's processed equivalent.

The first step is to remove the processed food. It will take a few weeks, but your tastes will adjust to the natural flavors as you remove the processed chemical concoctions from your palate. This isn't to say that you can't or will never have a processed food ever again. The goal is to re-set your taste preferences. The chemical flavorings are intended to overly excite your mind, leading you to overeat. Real food interacts with our bodies in ways that trigger our ability to interpret fullness. While an over-simplification of our biological processes, this serves to help us understand that our natural abilities are easily overridden by processed food. If confronted with heavily-flavored processed chips, I know that my tendency is to overeat. It's incredibly difficult to override a product that was made with the very intention of altering your body's ability to regulate your consumption. By focusing on real food, you enable your body's natural tendencies to beautifully serve you. You also eliminate a losing battle with willpower. It's not a good method for long-term health, and it can't serve you even short-term when faced with processed foods. We're meant to take pleasure in flavor-filled real foods. You tell me that a strawberry bursting with flavor in early spring doesn't bring a smile to your face. Life is threaded together by small and large moments of joy. I'm content with allowing a strawberry in peak season to bestow upon me one of those moments.

But if I'm being honest, I also love refried beans from a can. I sometimes don't even warm them up. Just an open can, a spoon, and me, leaning over the kitchen counter with a contented grin on my face. We oftentimes paint food pleasure as this elusive, unattainable future event, but it doesn't need to be. Food pleasure can take the shape of a garden dinner at a restaurant in the Tuscan hills as much as it can happen at your kitchen counter, eating a food you love out of a can. Don't let anyone tell you otherwise.

I would be remiss if I didn't address the fears that people hold around giving into food pleasure and I want to take a moment to address and honor them. Food addiction is a very real affliction, and the thought of taking pleasure in food is something that can instill the fear of never being able to stop. I have a dear friend who has battled food addiction her entire life, and she expressed to me the plight of the food addict:

"How do you love something that brings you such pain? It's also something you require. You can't avoid food. That's what makes this different from an addiction to alcohol. I can't just avoid going grocery shopping."

Alcoholics are advised to stay away from bars, but food addicts cannot avoid the source of their addiction. I won't portend that I'm an expert on food addiction, but I will refer back to chapter three where we discussed the holes in our lives and what we're trying to fill. Eating is an activity that we do three times a day, and denying oneself pleasure that many times a day will only serve to expand the rubber band of binge and restriction. It will catapult from one side to the other repeatedly, and eventually it will snap. When we exist for so long on the restrict side of the spectrum, our bodies are unsure when they will again receive a proper meal. The body has mechanisms to make us overeat in case food will again be scarce. When we slowly learn to trust our innate ability to feed ourselves, we build the capability to lean a bit more into the pleasures of the table, understanding that pleasure can come from a strawberry as much as it can come from a doughnut. We learn to expand our definition of food pleasure while learning how to care for the body with which we were entrusted.

Food pleasure is about enjoying our food as much as it's about the pleasures afforded us through the table. When asked about a special meal, people often talk about the activity around the table, sharing life through conversation and connection as well as through the experience of a shared meal. Food is inherently social. This social component feeds our souls in ways the food itself cannot. Lean into that.

CAN I FEED YOU?

Outside of San Sebastien, Spain, there is a one-Michelin-starred restaurant called Elkano. They are renowned for their turbot, which is simply seasoned and cooked over an open-charcoal grill, imparting a slight smokiness into the morning's catch. The restaurant sits in the tiny fishing village of Getaria. Elkano is family-owned and the chef, Aitor Arregui, took us to the fishing port and told us how they get their fish each morning and how they work with the fishermen to prevent over-fishing. He was not only a chef, but a protector of his family's tradition and the ocean that graciously provided the daily sustenance. He told us how he would run around the dining room as a little boy and learn the trade from his father. This restaurant was his home.

In the dining room, he would come over as each dish arrived and would excitedly detail what we were eating, how it was prepared, and how it showcased the natural beauty of the fish. He showed us how to grab the tail of a small fish and pull to extract the meat and leave the vertebrae behind. He displayed this technique for my side of the table and turned to me: "Can I feed you?" The answer to that question is always an unequivocal, "Yes!" He placed the fish in my mouth and explained all of the flavors I was experiencing.

The main dish was turbot, a flat fish with both eyes on the left side of its body. It has a light-skinned side and a dark-skinned side, as one side faces upward toward the sun and the bottom side receives little light. Aitor came over to our platter and explained the beautiful nuances of the flavor of the meat based on which side of the turbot it came. He asked our permission to show us something and proceeded to dig through our turbot with a fork, looking for the tiniest bone. He asked for a phone, turned on its flashlight, grabbed a water glass, and placed it upside-down over the phone's light. He then placed the tiniest bone on top and inspected it closely. "Come here! Closer! Look!" We had no idea what he was doing but his excitement was contagious. He pointed out the faintest of gray rings on the bone. "See the rings? This fish was three years old!"

We were dumbfounded. He had an astonishing amount of knowledge and respect for the fish in front of us and the sea from where it came. We could have devoured this fish and savored its flavor but were so close to missing this clue that hid inside. Aitor encourages all of his guests to eat with their hands. Michelin star or not, he believes that your hands are the best tools to fully experience every morsel of fish, especially the oft-missed pieces close to the bones. Eating was a sensory experience and it was his humble mission to instill this lesson in each person lucky enough to dine at Elkano. He left us to continue our meal and stare at the tiny bone positioned over a phone light and a glass. Five minutes prior, we had no idea that this tiny bone was hidden in our fish and would reveal the age of our meal.

I watched as he went from table to table and asked for permission to prod through their food and tell the story of it. The fish at Elkano remains some of the best I've had in my entire life, and I have a feeling it will be the best I'll ever have the honor of enjoying. The meal was spectacular, no doubt, but it was Aitor and his story and his passion that brought the simplest of meals to life. He embodied the metabolism of passion; he brought much knowledge and paired it with unbelievable pleasure. Joy emanated from his exuberance for his craft and what he could share with his guests. The days of a chef are long, but Aitor gave us much more than a meal that day; he showed us how knowledge and pleasure make for a beautiful food experience.

Food pleasure is not about indulgence. It's not about healthy or unhealthy foods. It's not about excess. It's about a deep understanding of the pleasures of the table and how they lead to life-long healthy relationships with food. Sometimes these pleasures look like a holiday meal; other times they look like a quickly fried egg over toast with sautéed greens. Pleasure can come from the knowledge that you made yourself a meal, even if it's as uninspiring as peanut butter and banana. It's about the ability to enjoy a pizza night with friends as much as it's about savoring a quick solo meal at home. Pleasure does not require the presence of inspiration. Habits that restore your relationship with food come from the daily interactions you have with the table, not just from the festive feasts. The more you learn to derive pleasure from the simple, the more you understand the table as a positive life-source.

Yes, we can and should talk about the chocolate cake, and eat it, too. Life's too short not to.

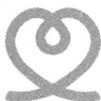

SUGGESTED PROJECT: SEEK THE PLEASURES OF THE TABLE

Virginia Woolf once said, "For pleasure has no relish unless we share it." Aim to share the pleasures of the table. With friends and/or family, plan a meal together with components that are meaningful to each person. It can be as simple as a pasta dinner with a side salad. Make your own sauce for the pasta and dressing for the salad. Keep it simple and fun. By making your own pasta sauce and salad dressing, you'll take two easily processed ingredients and turn them into real-food options. These are also two things that you can easily recreate on busy nights once you create the habit.

Make the table. We first eat with our eyes, so use the good plates and the cloth napkins. Pour the wine. Make a point of enjoying the conversations, the experience, and the meal.

After it's done, think about how it made you feel. Are you more relaxed? Stressed? Ask "Why?" numerous times to uncover the root of how this experience made you feel. How can you lean more often into the pleasures of the table?

Then, take these lessons into the next meal you make for yourself when you are eating at home alone. How can you create rituals around simple mealtimes? The beauty of food pleasure is that it can exist at a pasta dinner with friends as much as it can exist over a solo meal of a soft-boiled egg over a salad. The spectrum of food pleasure allows us to experience it in all of its forms at the table. Explore how you can incorporate this more readily into your life.

SECTION II:
UNDERSTANDING THE AMERICAN FOOD LANDSCAPE

"To know the food culture is to know the people's lives. To know the people's lives is to know the way people feel and think." [1]

SHOJIN RYORI PROJECT

Everything we hold as eaters must operate in a challenging food landscape. The table provides a meeting place for all that we are, and our food environment impacts the options available to us and the ease with which we come to the table.

CHAPTER 5

THE FIGHT FOR THE AMERICAN BREAKFAST TABLE

"The literature on obesity is not only voluminous, it is also full of conflicting and confusing reports and opinions. One might well add to this the words of Artemus Ward: 'The researches of so many eminent scientific men have thrown so much darkness on the subject that if they continue these researches we shall soon know nothing.'" [2]

HILDE BRUCH

Now that we have a better sense of who we are as eaters, let us turn our focus to the American food landscape. It's vital to understand how our food environment, and by further extension our society, impacts how we come to the table and even what is on our tables. We don't exist as eaters in a vacuum, and while that is to be celebrated, it brings with it its own challenges. The current American nutritional state is characterized by an obsession around labels and is more focused on what people are *not* eating than what they are.

"I'm giving up coffee."

"Oh! I've wanted to do that for so long!"

"Me? This month I'm cutting out gluten."

This reductive focus on foods isn't commonly seen outside of America. In many areas of the world, people eat familiar foods that are passed down throughout generations, and they feel connected to their families through the foods they eat. In the U.S., we've entered a phase where people focus more on their restrictions than the food they do eat and the nourishment it provides. I'm not opposed to experimenting to see what foods serve your body best, on the contrary, but we need to stop equating health with the level of our willpower to sustain a restrictive diet. That's not health, and it doesn't last. As we covered in the last section, we're grasping at straws, trying to fill a void that food can't fill. The times I have lived in Europe and travelled in Asia, I never heard such an unnatural emphasis placed on the foods people were not eating. In America, we wear our restricted foods list like a badge of honor. By refusing ourselves the pleasure of the table, we think ourselves stronger for it.

How we approach the table has been changed by a century of wars, as we'll examine shortly, that have shaped how we produce, distribute, and view food. America has long been a country of opposites and contradictions. Our current food culture of abundance has roots in its impoverished history of the Great Depression, and our overindulgence of food can be traced to our Puritan values that emphasized the denial of pleasure.[3] We have been conditioned to eat not what we enjoy, but instead to choose whichever recently popularized superfood promises health and longevity. Attention-grabbing nutrition headlines are happy to feed this hunger. Oddly enough, the American breakfast table most aptly captures this ever-changing nutritional guidance. We swing from bacon and eggs to cereals and muffins to avocado and back to bacon. In his seminal book, *Nutritionism*, Gyorgy Scrinis provides a framework of three distinct time periods in 20th century America that have shaped our current state of nutritional confusion.[4] Using this framework, we'll explore the trajectory of the American food system and the development of a damaged food culture.

LATE NINETEENTH CENTURY TO THE MID-TWENTIETH CENTURY

In the early twentieth century, the U.S. food supply started industrializing for a collection of reasons. Paving the way for the new industrialized food system were three important innovations: refrigerated rail cars, canning, and pasteurization.

Each of these served to extend the shelf life of foods and enable foods to travel farther distances. People were no longer limited to foods in their local areas and the practice of seasonal eating began its decline. As the distance that food traveled increased, so did the food choices available to the American public.[5]

Nutrition science at the turn of the century was led by the discovery of macros and micros. Food started to be seen through the lens of carbohydrates, proteins, fats, and vitamins. It is during this time that the American public received the message of eating for health rather than basing food decisions simply on what they enjoyed. As nutritional discoveries were made, nutrition scientists proposed drastic changes to the American diet with little evidence. Home economists, cookbook writers, and the marketing world also added to the nutritional frenzy. Eating no longer focused on sitting around the table with seasonal foods, and instead focused on understanding the nutritional breakdown of what was on the plate. The discovery of the calorie changed, even to the modern day, how we analyze our intake and burning of food for energy. The public quickly rallied around the idea that one must not consume more calories than it would be possible to burn off.[6] Food, health, and the body became quantifiable and nutrition became measurable. Due to the diseases of nutritional deficiencies, nutrition science focused on recommendations for consuming enough of the nutrients necessary to ward off those diseases. With the discovery of vitamins, the public believed that their food supply did not provide enough nutrients, a perception that permeates into the modern day.[7]

The caloric measurement provided an understanding of the food we eat in a way that disconnected us from the source. It did not provide information on the quality of the food, how it was produced, or how it was transformed through processing. As we will see through the analysis of some of the world's healthiest areas, they hold a deep understanding and knowledge of why they consume certain ingredients, how they are sourced, how they are produced, and why they eat them. The calorie provides none of this information. In fact, it cloaks the need to understand these attributes of our food supply. If a carrot calorie is equal to a calorie from industrially-produced meat, and nutrition is merely an equation of calories in versus calories out, then we no longer need to expend the mind space to understand these extraneous details. The calorie frees us of that burden, but the calorie does not capture how the body metabolizes the food differently. We are just beginning to understand how the nutrients in one plant work together for human health.[8] The symbiotic relationship of nutrients within our food, and how the body interprets and metabolizes them, have yet to be discovered. The calorie does not speak to either of these functions.[9] We continue to try to speak to the body in a language it does not understand.

The eating habits of Americans had been irrevocably shaped by the industrial food model from the start of the First World War, creating eating habits that would continue to be fed by the industrial model for the century to come. By the time the Great Depression hit in the 1920s, Americans were not sure that they would emerge unscathed. One-third of Americans did not have enough food during this time.[10] The act of standing in line for bread and an overwhelming sense of need characterized this generation for decades to come. My mother has dry spices in her pantry from the 1970s. When I ask her why she won't throw them away and replace them, she'll remark that she never knows when she'll need them. Even though she didn't grow up during the Great Depression, she was raised by a generation who did, and they instilled those lessons into the next generation. Interestingly, the finger of nutritional science began to place the blame of poor diets directly on people's ignorance. Dietitians and home economists blamed nutritional ignorance for the poor diets of low-income individuals instead of the poverty itself.[11]

World War II served to fully imprint the industrial food model on the American food system. The government worked with private businesses to concentrate efforts on winning the war. With the force of the American food system placed into this effort, the production and manufacturing of industrialized food accelerated. In the post-war period, the U.S. government worked with farmers and agriculture scientists to ensure there was enough food, both for Americans and for war-ravaged areas abroad. This need, combined with the growing global population, brought forth the Green Revolution, a period marked by the invention of engineered seeds to increase yields. Severe famines were predicted in the mid-1950s, with an estimated death toll of around one billion people as agriculture had reached its carrying capacity. Norman Borlaug, 1970 Nobel Peace Prize recipient, is considered the Father of the Green Revolution. An agriculturist by trade, Borlaug went to Mexico and bred wheat to evolve quickly and increase its output by around 70%.[12] As detailed in the research of Amy Bentley and Hi'ilei Hobart, this change in agriculture "put severe strain on local economies and endangered subsistence farmers, the environment, and indigenous cultures."[13] The post-war period transformed the need for industrial food from a temporary war-time effort to a permanent system to feed everyday Americans.[14]

The large-scale supermarket became a permanent part of America during this post-war period. The corner store, the butcher, and the baker receded into the landscape of American history, and the new supermarkets reflected the new American ideals of abundance. They become synonymous with what it means to be American.[15] The hunger and desperate sense of need of the Great Depression were still in the memories of many, enabling the supermarket to shine as a beacon of American ingenuity and perseverance. American tastes were also beginning to change as both soldiers and affluent American travelers returned home with changed tastes after experiencing European and other foreign foods. The American food landscape of the 1950s included a small number of world cuisines, but immigrants were still cooking their traditional foods at home, providing a bridge between their food cultures and that of their new home.[16]

THE CORNER STORE, THE BUTCHER, AND
THE BAKER

As humans, we crave connection. The sterile corners of the supermarket fail to provide this. In other places in the world, the food cornerstones of the corner store, the butcher, and the baker still exist and provide a connection between the people who produce or procure your food and you.

In Italy, I had "my" butcher around the corner. He was a stocky guy perhaps in his upper 30s, and always with a twinkle in his eye. He put up with my broken Italian with a smile and would help me select cuts of meat, especially when the cut of meat I needed (and had thus learned the corresponding Italian translation) wasn't available. Cuts of meat aren't the first words you learn in a foreign language, so I would look up the name of the cut and practice it as I walked to his shop. If he was out of that particular cut, then I needed to pivot quickly and learn how to ask for something comparable. I would attempt to explain what I was making, and he would help me understand which meat was best due to its fat content, muscle fiber, etc. These small exchanges brought light to my days and enabled me to share a pleasure of human existence with my butcher—the act of cooking and sharing dishes.

Masters of their crafts, like butchers and bakers, do not only sell their goods; their role is not one of mere transaction. They are able to delight in what you're purchasing and making with their goods. This made cooking seem like a communal activity. As I went back home time and time again after visiting him, I carried a piece of him and his knowledge with me back to the kitchen. I loved being able to get cooking tips and talk about the future meal I was planning with the very people from whom I purchased. These small moments of joy matter, and they matter deeply.

EARLY 1960S TO THE MID-1990S

This period in American food history was marked by the binary categorization of nutrients as either good or bad. Bred from this mentality were the moralistic food labels and thinking that permeate American society today. American doctors also turned to biomarkers as indicators of health, increasing the myopic lens of health and nutrition. As nutrient deficiencies became less common, the public health arena turned toward the prevention of chronic diseases through the analysis of whether nutrients were good and prevented disease or bad and contributed to it. This era was partly caused by the preceding decades' thinking when nutritional knowledge pushed the public to consume enough protective nutrients. This new era caused the nutritional lens once to once again shift as concern grew that the public might now be overconsuming. This concern, along with the concentration on biomarkers, spurred the national endeavor to reduce the amount of fat that Americans were consuming, a decision that shaped the American view of health and nutrition for decades to come.[17]

Healthy eating was defined as a conscious reduction of fat (with an emphasis on saturated fat), a focus on the consumption of complex carbohydrates and fiber, as well as shifting fat intake from saturated towards polyunsaturated fats. While nutrition scientists intended for these guidelines to steer us toward whole foods like beans and vegetables, the industrial food model was more than happy to fill the new need with low-fat cakes. As nutrition guidelines focused more on nutrients than on whole foods, it became increasingly easier to blur the line between real and processed foods. A nutrient-centric lens can make a low-fat industrial cake appear to be a better option than a natural nut butter on whole grain bread. The American public was told to remove fat from all foods, yet they were not educated on the difference between fats from real foods versus those in processed foods.[18] Stanley Ulijaszek detailed in "Evolving Human Nutrition" how the food industry can distort the nutritional needs of a population: "...the deep social embeddedness of food as a symbolic good is something that is actively exploited by food manufacturers and marketers, and can have profound effects on the nutritional health of populations."[19] The pursuit to reduce fat had profound effects on the American diet and were further cemented in U.S. dietary guidelines.

1977 was a pivotal year in twentieth-century American nutrition history, guided by Senator George McGovern's Senate Select Committee on Nutrition and Human Needs. Concerned about the rising rates of coronary heart disease, and pushed by the American Medical Association, the 1977 "Dietary Goals for the United States" emphasized the good/bad categorization of nutrients even further. The meat, dairy, and sugar lobbies greatly influenced the final version, fighting to avoid any language that specifically called for the reduced consumption of red meat, dairy, or sugar. By concentrating on nutrients, the Dietary Goals could appease the food lobbies by calling for an increased consumption of good nutrients (unsaturated fats and vitamins and antioxidants) while reducing our consumption of the bad ones (saturated fats, cholesterol, calories). This guidance took nutritional science and simplified it to the sum of its parts while complicating any chance of providing meaningful whole food guidance to the American public. Raymond Reiser, a nutrition scientist, called the advice to reduce saturated fat an "oversimplification of the science," but the groundwork had been laid for a reductionist view of nutrition paired with the cautionary advice to eat less.[20] The 1977 guidelines cemented the change in nutritional focus that started in the early 1960s from a whole food approach to that of a nutrient focus.[21]

Culinary interest began to change in the 1970s and 80s as there was an emergence of interest in the culinary arts, as well as the beginning of an appreciation for American indigenous foods. Housewives were influenced by Julia Child's "Mastering the Art of French Cooking" and Time-Life published a series of cookbooks called "Foods of the World" that became popular among the educated middle class. Some of these volumes discussed American indigenous foods, spurring a budding interest in the variety of foods offered at home. Additionally, historians and social scientists took an interest in food history, solidifying food as a serious focus for one of the first times by the early 1990s.[22] These counter-movements were small compared with the growing national frenzy around the reduction of fat, but their emergence started to pave the way for a new focus on food and nutrition.

MID-1990S TO THE PRESENT

This period of American history was characterized by the advancement of science into the role of nutrients on specific functions of the body. Scientists were able to molecularly analyze the effects of nutrients on the body. Nutrients were no longer only labeled as good or bad but were also tied to biomarkers and health conditions. Nutritional advice moved from a more negative outlook to a positive one, asserting that the increased consumption of protective nutrients was beneficial. Food and nutrients were tied to function, and the food system stepped in quickly with the emergence of new products touting their nutritional benefits as tied to bodily functions.[23]

A few fundamental changes from the previous era laid the groundwork for this period of nutrition. The guidance to consume low-fat was starting to be questioned and overturned, led by the discovery of trans-fats, found in so many of the golden foods of the low-fat era. Margarine, one of the highly promoted industrial foods during the low-fat years, fell from grace, leading to increased nutritional confusion in the public as a generation of Americans had only lived during the time of the low-fat campaign.[24] How could Americans know how to feed themselves when the only nutritional advice they had received was just turned on its head?

Functional nutrition, defined by Scrinis as the "targeted view of nutrients and foods as 'functional' in relation to bodily health," further distanced Americans from their food.[25] While they were analyzing their food myopically, they forgot to look up and see the whole picture. Fortified cereals labeled good for heart health were not seen as a processed food through the lens of functional foods. Nutrients mattered more than the actual ingredients or processing. Processing could be used to disguise lesser foods by adding nutrients and their associated health claims, and thus the food industry developed new ways to change the nutritional profile of food. In the search for the proper ratio of functional nutrients, Americans began to eat more. A varied diet could no longer meet their nutritional needs, so they sought out modified foods to satiate their nutrient hunger. When specific quantities of nutrients equal health, there is little room for error.[26]

This highlighted a big shift in how Americans received their nutritional information. In contrast to the importance of the 1977 Dietary Goals, Americans encountered nutritional data differently from the 1990s onward. Functional nutrients resonated with the American public, giving them a tangible way to eat their favorite foods while feeling like they were making healthy food decisions. The advice of nutrition experts became less important and visible as marketing departments of food companies were free to consume, distort, and convey nutritional studies in ways that promoted their nutritionally-adjusted products. These health claims became trusted sources from which Americans received their nutritional knowledge.[27]

The counter-movement of the 1980s gained momentum during the 1990s and 2000s, stimulated by the increasingly narrow view of food, nutrients, and health. Food studies emerged as a veritable academic course of study, placing food as a legitimate topic worthy of understanding. Through this study of food, scholars became aware of the interconnected nature of food, nutrition, the environment, flavor, conviviality, and other factors. Some of the early pioneers of this counter-movement were Alice Waters, Carlo Petrini, and Michael Pollan. They understood the interconnected nature of food and pushed for a transformed food system that acknowledges the roles of sustainability, nutrition, taste, and cultural factors.[28]

FUNCTIONAL NUTRITION IN THAILAND

In Thailand, food is seen as a life-source, and they understand how the food they eat directly correlates to bodily health. In my graduate program, I stayed with a family in a rural village in Phatthalung, Thailand. The grandmother and grandfather I stayed with were both elders of the village and were also healers. They used the plants, foods, and herbs of their surroundings to treat and heal members of the village. When we sat down to our first meal with the family, I was moved by how they painstakingly described each dish, not in terms of gastronomic contents, but in its ability to aid the body.

"This chicken curry contains the plant that is growing by the fence over there. Do you see it? It helps with the milk production of new mothers."

This continued as each dish was described by the ingredients that supported the body. I happened to be staying with the village healers, and the medicinal garden in their yard was a source for many additions to the food they made.

The next day we attended a rice festival with the entire village and we had the opportunity to cook with the villagers. Again, dish after dish was explained with what was in it, how to process it into the dish (e.g. pound in a mortar and pestle, chop, etc.), and how it supported the body. It wasn't uncommon to hear, "Chop this leaf that supports the respiratory system with the garlic," and, "This herb is good for the liver."

Unlike American culture, the ingredients they described were all real food ingredients from their local surroundings. They weren't described in terms of their vitamin content and how that nutritional make-up was then added to processed foods. No, they used the ingredients in their natural form, described how they benefited the body, and enjoyed the dishes with pleasure.

THE IMPACT OF NUTRITIONISM

"As for butter versus margarine, I trust cows more than chemists."

JOAN GUSSOW[29]

Gyorgy Scrinis defines nutritionism as the "reductive focus on the nutrient composition of foods as the means for understanding their healthfulness, as well as by a reductive interpretation of the role of these nutrients in bodily health."[30] We've examined how nutritionism developed over twentieth-century America; we will now turn our focus to see how this has shaped the way Americans view food and come to the table. Nutritionism, by separating us from our food source, greatly differentiates our habits from some of the world's healthy food cultures. Nutritionism extends beyond the scientific understanding of our food. Its wide reach and damage is found in the application of the scientific studies to guide how our food is marketed, engineered, and labeled. It is through these latter avenues that the nutritional messages reach the public, and these are the avenues they ultimately turn to and trust.[31]

In the pursuit of the perfect plate, Americans turned to experts to dictate what should be on it. Meanwhile, Americans were largely not aware of the disagreements within the nutritional community. Scientists still have much to discover to deepen their understanding of how the food we eat and our health are interconnected, yet the industry could easily mask those disagreements and the advancements still to be made by only choosing to highlight research that supported their products. Scientific discoveries over the twentieth century have revealed that the web of food and health is incredibly intricate. The varying amount of vitamin A in food provides the perfect example of the intricacies of our food. According to the National Institutes of Health, "RDAs [Recommended Dietary Allowance] for vitamin A are given as mcg of retinol activity equivalents (RAE) to account for the different bioactivities of retinol and provitamin A carotenoids."[32] Three ounces of fried beef liver contain 6,582 mcg RAE (444% of our recommended daily value) while 64 grams of chopped raw carrots contain 459 mcg RAE (184% of our recommended daily value), yet the body knows how to metabolize these varying ranges.[33] How amazing is our body? Nutritionism ignores the complexity of our food and says that we can eat a certain fortified food to reduce our risk of heart disease.[34] It also serves to mask how the processing of foods and additives can greatly change the nutritional content of a whole food.

Throughout the twentieth century, nutritional confusion persisted. The American public, facing increasing rates of heart disease, was told to avoid or reduce their consumption of eggs, due to the cholesterol found in the yolk. This had the effect of changing the American breakfast table to include processed and fortified breakfast cereals. Gone were the whole eggs, along with the butter. Margarine perfectly illuminates the change from traditional wisdom and whole foods to that of a reductive approach to food.[35] In 1984 Time magazine published its cover with a picture of two fried eggs forming eyes and an upside down curved bacon slice forming the sad mouth of a face. The issue was entitled, "Cholesterol: And Now the Bad News".[36] Thirty years later, an artistically swirled piece of butter graced the cover of the 2014 edition of Time magazine, entitled, "Eat Butter: Scientists labeled fat the enemy. Why they were wrong".[37] People had lived almost all of their lives under this mistaken advice. The American public had taken to heart the advice of nutritional scientists (and fallen victim to how the findings were conveyed), and this changed decades of eating habits.

Human engagement with food is severed through the nutritionism lens. Nutritionism created a population dependent upon nutritional scientists and nutritional research to understand how to feed themselves.[38] When this failed, how were they to know what to put on the table? A reductive approach had taught them that there is no difference between beef and a highly processed piece of beef jerky. The pervasive logic that a "protein is a protein" convinced the public that the body would metabolize both in the same way. Nutritionism steered Americans away from seeing whole foods as having all the nutrition they required. It took their traditional knowledge and said, "That's no longer valid. You need to understand the latest nutritional discoveries." As Scrinis detailed in *Nutritionism*, "The authority of traditional and cultural knowledge of food, or of people's own sensual and practical experience with food, has been correspondingly devalued."[39] By understanding food at the nutrient level, Americans formed distant and misconstrued relationships with their food. This is largely because humans have historically eaten food with cultural underpinnings, not combinations of nutrients devoid of tradition; and this food is intended to be eaten together, shared around a table. Nutritionism separated Americans from the processes of growing, preparing, and enjoying food.[40] This created a chasm so deep that Americans lost their ability to eat intuitively, guided by tradition and the wisdom of previous generations. The ill-health that came with the processed foods brought about a frenzy around the metabolism of weight-loss, instead of an understanding of the importance of food enjoyment and knowledge of the food that is placed on the table. Food became a precise equation waiting to be solved, instead of a place where one finds enjoyment.[41]

Spurring the focus on weight loss was the nutrient transition that occurred in the twentieth century. The changes in food, physical activity (due to the advent of easier methods of transportation that reduced the amount we walk), and the decline in health changed the nutritional landscape. Society previously had faced high-levels of famine and malnutrition, directly causing an increase in infectious diseases. Additionally, daily work had been largely labor-intensive. In the twentieth century, we experienced a shift in work from labor-intensive to less labor-intensive technology-based work. This decrease in physical activity was coupled with the change in diet to more processed foods. Malnutrition became less of a public health epidemic and, in the 1980s and 90s, the prevalence of infectious diseases switched to an increase in diet-related non-communicable diseases across the world. The diet-related diseases of obesity and diabetes became pervasive problems in low-to-middle-income countries in the world.[42] We see this in the United States today as the rates of obesity disproportionately affect people living in low-income areas. While the nutrition transition did serve to reduce infectious diseases and extend life expectancy, there is clearly another stage to be pursued. Barry Popkin details this third stage as one of behavioral change where the public eats more fruits and vegetables (i.e. whole foods) and increases its level of physical activity, thus decreasing body mass.[43] I would add to this stage that, in the case of Americans, they must repair their relationship with food through an increased understanding of how their food is produced, sourced, and processed. The challenge in properly addressing the nutrition transition is that the change incorporated an increase in the consumption of fats and sugars and salts, all pleasurable tastes to humans. Sugar, in particular, has been shown to be an addictive substance.[44] The sweet flavor is also an early indicator of energy to infants, emphasizing how early the sweetness reward system is developed.[45]

The increase in obesity due to the changes in diet, and the call by the government to reduce caloric consumption, led to an increased focus on caloric intake. It is important to note the role that this caloric reductionism had on the American relationship with food. Caloric reductionism taught Americans that one-hundred calories of a reduced-fat highly-processed cookie were the same as one-hundred calories of an apple. This intense focus on calories helped to nurture the processed food rise in America, as 100-calorie packs of America's favorite processed foods filled grocery store shelves, promising satiation without sacrificing the waistline. Caloric reductionism does not even begin to address how the body metabolizes different foods. It furthers the misplaced logic that we can place a precise number on the body's nutritional needs. The difference with the focus on calories is that nutrients are part and parcel of the food, but calories are an external measurement, providing no indication as to the processing level of the food. Nutrition science is beginning to investigate how the body metabolizes processed foods (e.g. trans-fat) differently from whole foods. It is also starting to uncover how one body to the other metabolizes the same food in different ways.[46] This cannot be captured completely in a scientific food-health equation.

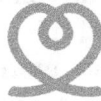

SUGGESTED PROJECT: SEEK OUT THE CONFUSION

For the next week or two, pay attention to the nutritional guidance you hear and see, both in the news and at the grocery store, and you're bound to find contradictory advice. Using the same strategy learned in Chapter 3, approach this with amusement and curiosity. Instead of giving nutritional news the power to make you feel crazy, separate yourself from it. See how often you see nutritionism at play in the grocery store. Unprocessed foods like broccoli and oranges don't advertise themselves as healthy because they don't need to, but the middle rows of processed foods will always tout their health claims. Become familiar with how nutritionism exists in your world. Question everything and ask, Does this actually make sense to me? Do a gut check with this each step of the way. The more you familiarize yourself with the nutritional world in which you live, the more you're able to see through the ploys and establish an intuitive sense of health.

CHAPTER 6
THE INGREDIENTS OF HEALTHY FOOD CULTURES

I have laid out the trajectory of nutrition history in twentieth century America and analyzed how nutritionism negatively impacted Americans' relationships with food and health by pulling them farther from their food source. Through this transition, the United States has developed an unhealthy food culture that becomes increasingly difficult to alter. However, there are numerous anthropological studies into the inner-workings of the world's healthiest food cultures. In these areas, their traditional knowledge guides how they choose their foods, how they come to the table, and how they live.[1] I will examine a few of these healthy areas, detail what is on their table and how they come to the table, and analyze what sets them apart from the current food culture in America.

When experts analyze health, they look at both life-expectancy and the years of end-of-life morbidity. Morbidity is defined as a diseased state or ill health.[2] Dan Buettner led a team from National Geographic to explore the world's healthiest areas with the longest-lived peoples, dubbed the "Blue Zones" by Buettner and his team. His studies brought him to Okinawa, Japan; Lomo Linda, California; Ikaria, Greece; Nicoya, Costa Rica; and Sardinia, Italy. Okinawans have less dementia, cancer, and heart disease than Americans, and they have the longest morbidity-free life expectancy in the world. In Lomo Linda, California, the Seventh-day Adventist church was founded in the 1840s. The church and its members view health as part of their faith. This community lives up to a decade longer than other Americans. In Nicoya, Costa Rica, a sixty-year-old is four times more likely to live to ninety than a sixty-year-old in the U.S. Moving to the Mediterranean, Sardinia contains ten times the number of centenarians than America. On Ikaria, the elderly population rarely suffers from the age-related diseases of dementia. Additionally, one-third of Ikarians live into their nineties.[3] The question then follows: how are they living and what are they eating that so drastically differentiates their health from that of other Americans? Furthermore, can America adapt some of these lessons to revolutionize how we come to the table?

WHAT'S ON THE TABLE

"Spread before us were plates of fresh fish, black-eyed peas with fennel, Greek salad, sourdough bread, and local wine—food that radiated health." [4]

Dan Buettner used these words to describe his lunch with Antonia Trichopoulo of the University of Athens in Ikaria, Greece. Dan asked her how he could convince the American population to eat real food like the spread in front of them. He had expected Trichopoulo to detail the nutritional benefits of the Greek foods as a way to persuade Americans. Instead, she responded with, "Feed them!"[5] Throughout all the Blue Zones you find a diet focused on an abundance of fruits and vegetables. Only Loma Linda, California contained a population of vegetarians. For those Seventh Day Adventists who consumed meat, the meat served as a side dish and not the main offering. It decorated the plate rather than overtaking it. This trend is also seen in the other Blue Zones. While all the other Blue Zone areas consumed meat, they consumed it sparingly, typically for some cause or celebration. Okinawans consumed some pork but only did so for occasional ceremonies, and even then, only in small quantities. Sardinians ate meat predominately on Sundays and some special occasions. The Blue Zones research did not reveal if the health of the studied populations was because of their meat consumption, or if their diets contained elements that overrode the negative impact of the meat. Nutritionism and reductive thinking will continue to try to answer this question, but the lesson from the Blue Zones is that meat, if consumed, should be done in moderation; and furthermore, it should be enjoyed.[6]

Blue Zone populations do not count their calories, nor do they take supplements or analyze their intake ratio of protein to carbohydrates. Food is central at celebratory occasions and, except for Lomo Linda, they consume wine moderately. Their focus on food is far from reductive and their health is directly tied to the foods they consume. All of these locations have plant-based diets and can easily access fruits and vegetables, if they don't grow their own. If they need to buy fruits and vegetables, then they know where to procure them for cheaper than the processed foods. Okinawans consume significant amounts of tofu, miso, and seaweed while Nicoyans combine fortified maize and beans for many of their meals, a food combination that is recognized as being nutritionally complementary. Ikarians eat a version of the Mediterranean diet with fruits, vegetables, beans, potatoes, whole grains, and olive oil. Sardinians also consume a Mediterranean-based diet of whole grain, beans, vegetables, fruits, and pecorino cheese from grass-fed sheep.[7] While their foods differ and reflect their individual cultures and the lands from which they live, they all contain whole foods. Traditional foods tend to be minimally processed and the combination of food, like that of the maize and beans in Nicoya, oftentimes increases the healthfulness of the individual foods. Nutrition science has not yet uncovered exactly how these food combinations produce a healthier dish than the individual ingredients alone, yet they have sustained generations.[8]

While Americans tend to focus on the food on the table, people in the Blue Zones also understand the importance of their agricultural practices, where their food is sourced, how the animals are raised, and the locality of their produce. There is a lack of appreciation for this level of understanding within the nutritional science community, but if we learn from the mistakes of nutritionism then we would know not to always wait for expert advice for what should be on our tables when traditional knowledge can fill that gap.[9]

Blue Zones populations have recipes to make their healthy food taste good. They understand that food should be delicious. Otherwise, you won't continue to eat it.[10] John Frank, Chair of Public Health Research at the University of Edinburgh studied the rapid rise in obesity in the U.S., England, Australia, Mexico, and Canada, and the comparatively slower growth in obesity in Switzerland, Italy, Spain, South Korea, and France. He surmised that the latter group partially experienced a slower rise in obesity because of their stronger traditional foods, whereas the English-speaking countries have cuisines that are recognized as being blander. Processed food brought with it more flavor in the form of fat, salt, and sugar, and the people in the countries with a relatively more bland cuisine embraced the new foods.[11] Processed foods contain higher amounts of salt and sugar than we find in whole foods, making them both more desirable and devoid of more nutrients.[12] Can a flavorful, traditional cuisine provide a level of resistance to the influx of processed foods? The Blue Zones seem to indicate that it is entirely possible.

With this information, what should be on the table? The obvious answer is whole foods that our body recognizes. Nutritionism made us question our food sources and break down whole foods to only eat the healthy parts, but residents in the Blue Zones don't analyze their food in that way. They eat the whole egg, not just the whites for fear of the cholesterol in the yolk. They don't remove the fat from their yogurts and cheeses. They don't attempt to nutritionally alter their foods, nor do they consume supplements. If food can provide health, then it can also provide all the necessary vitamins and minerals. Instead, residents in the Blue Zones utilize the traditional technique of fermentation not only to preserve their foods but also to make more nutrients available to the body. These Blue Zone societies use their local surroundings to provide seasonal ingredients that they honor through time-tested preparations.[13] Those are the dishes that make their way to the table.

HOW THEY COME TO THE TABLE

Convivial: relating to, occupied with, or fond of feasting, drinking, and good company[14]

Blue Zone communities understand the importance of the social fabric that connects them. This connectedness is a theme that runs throughout their lives, both at and away from the table. Blue Zones residents build strong social networks in their communities. Nicoyans are often visiting friends and family, if not living with their children or grandchildren. This injects a sense of purpose into their everyday existence. The Sardinian family unit is strong, and people know they are looked after. Science has been able to show us that a healthy family unit can lead to decreased rates of stress and depression. In Okinawa, the people form *moai*, a life-long group of friends who provide friendship, company, financial and emotional support.[15] This reduces stress as Okinawans know they have people who will support them throughout their lives. Scientists have searched for biomarkers to indicate why social connectedness has such an impact on our health and longevity. While they haven't been able to find the biomarkers, we inherently know that it matters. Spending time with people who care about you makes for a richer—and healthier—life.[16]

Blue Zone communities have movement as a natural part of their everyday lives. They don't lift weights or run marathons. Instead, they walk, garden, and simply move. Dan Buettner recorded this finding in the *Blue Zones Solution*: "None of the 253 spry centenarians I've met went on a diet, joined a gym, or took supplements. They didn't pursue longevity; it simply ensued."[17] Exercise was not a negative word or something they did for weight loss or increased muscle mass. Natural movement enables the Okinawans to garden, sit down and get up off the tatami mats numerous times a day. The Sardinian shepherds walk around five miles a day. The Ikarians could also be found gardening and walking to neighbors' houses. Even those in Loma Linda incorporated regular exercise into their daily activities. By having movement built into their lives and not something extra to make time for, it proved to be a daily habit. They also avoided the injuries that come from intense forms of exercise like running. The Adventist Health Survey found that marathon running is not required for a longer life expectancy. Regular, low-intensity exercise like walking reduces the risk of heart disease and some cancers.[18] Their lives emanated a sense of ease and flow, proving that exercise need not be a daily battle to achieve health and wellness.

This flow carried over into how they physically came to the table. As opposed to an American mentality of following a diet, actively trying to eat healthily, or indulging with guilt, the world's healthiest people come to the table with joy and grace. The elder Okinawans say a phrase before each meal, *hara hachi bu*, which loosely means to eat until you are eighty percent full. It takes the mind about twenty minutes to register a feeling of fullness, so eating until you are eighty percent full allows for the mind to register that you've had enough. This keeps them conscious of their intake so that they do not over-tax their systems with overconsumption. Instead of dieting, they have a sense of the proper amount needed by the body. By incorporating a saying or grace before a meal serves as a reminder that the food before you is special and should be treated in such a way. By placing more value on food, you change your relationship with it. It is difficult to express gratitude before a meal and consume low-quality food in a fast manner. Giving thanks forces you to pause and evaluate your meal in a different light.[19]

Communal dining also serves to add joy and meaning to the dining experience. How you eat is just as important as what you eat. All the Blue Zones emphasized communal dining, and people imitate what they see in the culture around them.[20] Just as a saying like *hara hachi bu* or grace before dinner reminds you that the event is special, so does the simple act of sharing food around a table. The Italian meal, in particular, provides an alternative to the rushed lives led by numerous Americans. A communal meal reminds you to slow down and savor both the food and the conversations around it. Industrial food is in stark contrast to the communal, slower meal because it enforces the belief that we don't have time for food—or with the sourcing of it or the act of cooking it. Industrial food can rid us of the problem of feeding ourselves.[21] However, Blue Zone communities don't see food as a problem from which to be freed. Instead, it is viewed as a punctuation to their days that provides nourishment and conviviality.

SINGLE-MINDED FOCUS

In Tsuruoka, Japan I visited Zenpo-ji temple and participated in meditation training. A Zazen Buddhist monk taught us how to position our body properly to align the spine and calm the mind. After meditation, we ate as the monks eat—in silence so as to absorb the energy of the food. He trained us to eat with the right posture of the heart. The food we were to receive was prepared by the hands of many people and we were to eat with gratitude for the energy of the food in front of us. We were to eat to receive the good energy from the food and to let that energy connect us to our soul. Our soul is contained in a body that is only ours, so we were to respect our body and that of the people who made our food. The food makes both the soul as well as the physical body. His teachings embodied an understanding of the sanctity of eating, and how it extended beyond the plate.

LESSONS FROM THE BLUE ZONES

A myopic view of the Blue Zones lessons leads us to analyze the precise foods eaten by the Okinawans in the hope to understand their functional attributes, but I believe this misses a fundamental outcome of the Blue Zones research: all Blue Zones areas have fundamentally different food cultures and foods, yet they are all flourishing. The attempt to import specific foods for American health negates the impact of the food culture that consumes them. People eat foods with flavors that are familiar through time-honored dishes influenced by their culinary traditions, around a table with friends and family. We tend to venerate the foods of other cultures without an appreciation for the whole foods that are present in our own lands. We need to acknowledge the wisdom of traditional foods without mistakenly thinking that we must also consume the specific foods from foreign lands. Health ensues when people stop their consumption of processed foods and eat traditional foods, and we have seen from the Blue Zones that traditional food varies from place to place. Perhaps the health benefits are due to the consumption of whole foods and not a specific traditional diet.[22] There is no single explanation for the health and longevity of the people in the Blue Zones, but upon examination we clearly see that how they come to the table becomes just as important as what is on the table.

Willpower is a finite muscle and, like any muscle, it eventually gives out. When we try to exercise the muscle of healthy eating and exercise, we overlook the ease with which we could be eating and living healthfully. What Dan and his team found was a network of healthy philosophies, including conviviality, daily exercise, and a sense of purpose. Food was the connective tissue by not only forming bonds around the table, but also providing a philosophy around how they interact with each other, their food, and themselves.[23] Our decisions about what to eat numerous times a day provide a framework for how we understand our relationship with food and the body.[24] The act of eating holds a special power, and until we recognize that, we will fail to make meaningful changes in our health and nutrition. In the words of Buettner, "For them, growing, preparing, serving, and eating are all sacred practices with the power to bring their families, their homes, their communities, their beliefs, and the natural world, together in daily rhythms and harmonies."[25] When these activities are in harmony, there is an ease with which you approach each of them.

This begs the question: how do you internalize these lessons in a society that is so entrenched in an industrial and processed relationship with food? Hawaii has been attempting to answer this question. Hawaii has a deep history of indigenous food and a recent history in the twentieth century with a highly processed food supply, as well as the health problems that come with it. Kauila Clark, a traditional healer and chairman of the board of a local Hawaiian medical clinic, has been working to encourage Hawaiians to eat healthier. He recognized the power of the marketing engine in pushing people to eat processed and fast foods. If he wanted people to change their deeply ingrained eating habits, he needed to find a way to reach Hawaiians at a deeper level than even the marketing giants. He did this through the power of a story:

> "I needed to find a story that would take people totally out of that realm so they could see that the issue of diet is something greater than themselves, something that also pays tribute to their ancestors...These [indigenous] foods are the foods that have ensured that you are here. You are a survivor in your family—your people made it for thousands of years on these foods, and you, right now, are the continuing link. What can you do to respect this process?"[26]

When processed food is readily available and enticing, you need to change the dialogue.[27] Touting the nutritional profile of foods is not a long-lasting technique for changing habits. When we understand that food is more than nourishment—it is people and connection—then we start to understand that a deeper story needs to be explored and told.

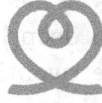

SUGGESTED PROJECT: ESTABLISH YOUR OWN BLUE ZONE

How can you incorporate the lessons from the Blue Zones, both at and away from the table? Start small and select one or two ways to incorporate healthy practices into your life that you want to try.

Examples to try:

- Take a walk with a friend

- Make a habit of eating one meal a day with others, enjoying the conviviality you can experience at the table

- Host a Sunday potluck with some of your favorite foods and people

- Add one vegetable to your meal

- Make time to have a glass of wine with friends one evening

Make sure they feel like something you *want* to embody, not something you feel like you *should*. As always, proceed with amusement and curiosity.

CHAPTER 7

EAT THIS AND THEN

Because Life Needs Frosting

Food marketing is genius. Let's just acknowledge that. Why? Because food marketing does what nutritional guidance fails to—it addresses who we are as eaters and it tells us a story. Unfortunately, it paints a story that entices us to purchase products attached with a promise of providing something in life that we believe we're in need of. *Because life needs frosting* is a ubiquitous pastry shop's tagline, responsible for the enticing aroma of cinnamon and sugar that perfumes numerous airports and shopping malls.

Companies know that we don't make the decision to buy a pastry out of knowledge of the ingredients. We make our purchasing decisions from the place where emotions meet the table. *Eat this and then you'll be happy. Eat this and then you'll be satiated. Eat this and then your life will be better.* Their marketing taps right into that. *Life is hard. This dessert makes it a little sweeter.* This is the story we're sold along with the pastry. However, we don't perceive that we're purchasing the story, even though the promise of "and then" remains in the front of our minds. The following table provides examples of food taglines from 2018 that tap into a deeper story, along with my interpretation of them.

TAGLINE	BEHIND THE TAGLINE
Have a Break	You're working hard and you deserve a break. This treat provides the break that you need and enables you to enjoy it more thoroughly.
It Gives You Wings	The pace of life is fast, and you need something to give you a bit of an edge and more courage to get through it. This provides the needed energy you require.
Breakfast of Champions	We hear time and time again how breakfast is the most important meal of the day. Champions and winners start their days with this breakfast. You want to be a champion, don't you?
Gather 'Round the Good Stuff	Pizza companies understand the conviviality of pizza. Pizza makes people think of the enjoyment of social occasions, sports games, and celebrations. This slogan makes pizza the focal point of these events.
Come Hungry, Leave Happy	This explicitly states the correlation between eating and happiness. The implication is that your hunger will not be the only thing satiated.
Eat Fresh	As America became more concerned with health, companies positioned themselves as a healthy alternative. Subconsciously they were telling people that choosing this food was a decision they need not feel guilty about.

Our inner dialogue drives many of our eating and purchasing decisions. Before I made the decision to leave my corporate job and pursue my passion for food in Italy, I distinctly remember sitting on my bed and observing the contents of my closet. Hanger upon hanger of expensive suits and heels of every color and style lined the shelves. In that moment, I realized that I had unsuccessfully attempted to buy my happiness to rid myself of the inner knowing that I was unfulfilled. This moment of clarity allowed me to release the power of my possessions. By creating space where there was previously none, I allowed for the exploration of the root of being at peace. I purposefully do not use the word *happy* because happiness implies a state of bliss, and that is not always attainable or desirable. Why? Most, if not all, of my growth comes from times where I've had to persevere with a tenacity I previously didn't embody. These moments of true grit enabled me to better understand my path, my voice, and my strength. I wouldn't characterize these periods of my life as times of happiness as we conventionally understand the word. Yet, I would not be who I am without them, and for that I'm eternally grateful. When we make a decision from the inner space of knowing, when we allow that tiny voice to speak, and when we create space for the unknown, we achieve a sense of ease and peace with our path, even when troubles arise. Because they will. Every good decision has always been met with struggles. In my corporate career, I always felt that the world around me dictated my life and my decisions. The long hours, the expectations, and the lack of work/life balance all created an ecosystem that held the puppet strings, controlling my every move. Once I set out on my path to own my decisions and my direction in life, I was better able to deal with the trying times that came, from the unknown financial situation and not knowing when my next paycheck would arrive, to the bureaucracy of picking up my life and moving to a foreign country. These were all the trials that came with my good decision. I found myself more than willing to work through them because they were challenges on my path, a path of my choosing.

My life didn't need frosting, at least not the kind that came in pastry form. By investing in the work of getting to the root of my unhappiness, I also freed myself from the call of consumerism. I tell you this personal anecdote because of the power of our inner dialogue, the power of the story we tell ourselves, and the story of ourselves that we allow others to place over our lives. Food marketing's power lies in its ability to tell us that we need something or are deserving of something. It seems counter-intuitive to say that we aren't worthy of something. The difference lies in our ability to understand the lie behind their promise and to understand our actual worth. My life does need frosting, but that frosting is found in the friendships I hold dear, the family that embraces me in love, and the real food in which I take pleasure and enjoy around a table with those I love most. As much as I've tried, I cannot and do not wish to do life alone. The frosting I add to my life is long-lasting and also embodies the lessons from those who live the longest in the Blue Zones. My frosting empowers me, holds me when I need it most, and, most importantly, makes my life one worth-living.

Food marketing can't hold a candle to that, try as they might. Life is constantly evolving, as it should. One week your frosting might actually be a cookie baked by a friend and enjoyed over conversation; another, it might be a well-needed day of rest from the chaos of the day-to-day; and yet another it might be popcorn in bed over your favorite movie. It's not a bad thing to have our frosting occasionally be food when we do the work of understanding why and how. We are dynamic beings who need to bring the conscious to the subconscious, time and time again. It's OK. In fact, it's more than OK. We should delight in this ability of ours to reshape, reform, and reclaim our relationship to ourselves and to the table. By bringing our consciousness to acts that were previously done with our subconscious, we build the ability to understand our actions and our motivations behind them. Food manufacturers desire that we stay in the subconscious, a place far more susceptible to marketing ploys. Part of reclaiming our relationship to ourselves and to the table is to turn marketing on its head and take every opportunity at the table to better understand who we are as eaters.

We allow for outside factors to shape our identity, both as eaters and as entities. This is why I advocate first for an understanding of our identities as eaters and ourselves, at and away from the table. When we do the work to know our identity—truly know and understand—then we are less susceptible to outside influences. We then bring this knowledge with us to the table. The siren call of marketing is watered down and less potent. We release its grasp. I know my food identity and I know that I don't need your product to provide frosting, or to make me happy, or any of the other seemingly endless calls of the food industry. This is why I advocate for understanding who we are as eaters first and foremost. We need to do the work of understanding our food identities and all that we bring to the table. Food marketing depends upon our willingness to outsource our identity. It may be a billion-dollar industry, but they are wrong to doubt our ability to self-identify and self-determine who we are, and who we want to be.

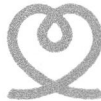

SUGGESTED PROJECT: DIG BENEATH THE MARKETING

For the next few days, pay attention to the food marketing around you. What speaks to you? What doesn't? Bring the conscious to the previously subconscious. When food marketing speaks to you, aim to understand why. In the case of a pastry shop, if a sweet treat that brings some frosting into your life sounds appealing, ask yourself, "Why?" Aim to understand what you're actually in need of. It's OK if your answer is that you simply want a pastry. This goal of this activity is to not talk yourself out of your feelings but to better understand the root of them and how food marketing plays to them. This is similar to the work we discussed in Chapter 3. By understanding what your "hole" is, you free yourself of the lies of food marketing. Take what you learned about the language of your body and aim to understand how food marketing taps into that language and the valid desires you have. Understand this connection and how to free yourself from it by paying attention to what you need.

CHAPTER 8

SUSHI, NOT FISH STEW

"Leisure is only possible when we are at one with ourselves. We tend to overwork as a means of self-escape, as a way of trying to justify our existence."

JOSEF PIEPER[1]

I'd be remiss if I didn't address the current state of corporate culture in America as it greatly impacts how we view the table and the frenzy with which we come to it. Lack of time and stress are often cited as leading examples for why we can't cook at home as much as we would like. Most of my clients are passionate women with full-time jobs, grad school classes, and a young one at home. They really do try to do it all, and finding time is oftentimes their first challenge. The fallacy of time is something we need to address from the start. I'm not minimizing the struggle to find enough time in your day. In fact, it's the opposite. I hold my clients in the highest esteem and greatly admire their tenacity. I, myself, struggled with finding time to cook when I was traveling extensively for work and working seventy-hour work weeks. Can we allow it to be alright that sometimes we can't cook? Can we allow ourselves the freedom and the space to stop aiming for one-hundred percent home-cooked?

Good. By creating this space, we can better address the fallacy of time. We make time for all kinds of priorities, from children to spouses to jobs. However, the very thing that enables us to care for our children, love our spouse, and tend to our job is the very body in which we dwell. Our inner dialogue is driven by how we feel about ourselves; our energy levels are impacted by the food we consume and the self-care we pursue; the health of our bodies directly impacts our ability to interact with the world around us and to positively impact what and whom we love. Somehow, we still don't value this dwelling of ours enough to prioritize its care.

The frenzy of our lives in America tells us a story of progress and perseverance, of tenacity and fortitude, yet it doesn't address the simple joy of the table and of investing in ourselves. By carving out time in our days to address the very task of feeding and caring for ourselves, we subconsciously tell ourselves that we're worthy of time and care. The narrative of corporate America tells us we should be at our best and always ready to perform, on little sleep and with even smaller amounts of nourishing food. When productivity equals self-worth, we become beings more concerned with doing than being. I would often walk around my office and ask people how they were. More often than not I was met with the following reply:

Great! Busy!

When did busyness become our identity? When did we allow the amount we produce to define our state of being? When you ask someone how they are in Arabic, you pose the question, *Kayf haal-ik*? Loosely translated, you are asking, *How is your heart doing at this moment*? How beautiful is that? How is your heart doing? How is your soul?[2] I don't want to know how busy you are and the frantic pace by which you define yourself. I'm not asking what you checked off your to-do list today. That likens you to a robot, whose existence is substantiated by the tasks accomplished and the accuracy by which they were done. I want to know your state of being. I want to know how you feel. I want to know what you're struggling with today, what you've overcome, and what gives you light for tomorrow.

Busy does not embody this. It doesn't even come close. In a society that is defined by our state of doing, it's no wonder that we see things like sleep, self-care, and making time to cook and enjoy our food as pleasures in which we can't indulge. Until we see them as an integral part of who we are as human beings, then we will fall victim to the fallacy of time. A person whose worth is determined by her daily accomplishments will not make time for frivolous extras until she reframes those extras as quintessential parts of who she is and when she allows these additions to align with her identity. They support her ability to pursue her passions each and every day. Busyness and burnout make for woeful friends in corporate America. We wear our lack of sleep and our ability to produce like badges of honor. We must reclaim our relationship to ourselves if we desire to fight the fallacy of time. Once we determine that our worth is not found in our doing, but in our being, then we can begin the real work of finding time in our days to nourish ourselves.

FAST FOOD IN JAPAN

During my month-long research in Japan, I was most struck by their fast food culture. In Japan, they consider sushi to be a fast food. The original sushi was fermented and took weeks, if not months, to be ready. By adding vinegar to the rice, they were able to add a fermented taste and turn sushi into a fast food. When I conducted interviews in Japan about their food culture, my Japanese interviewees spoke of fast food, but were referencing sushi or ramen, and soups with a proper *dashi* (Japanese stock) and nutritional value. Busy train stations in Japan are filled with real food alternatives, from soba to udon to sushi to bento boxes. It has been difficult for certain American fast food chains to gain a strong foothold in Japan because they have a local fast food culture that reflects the flavors of the region. If you take a look at the bento boxes across Japan, you'll find a regional representation of the food contained within.

Some companies are trying to take the fast food culture even further to not include any additives or preservatives, like Meat Delica Kudo company in Tsuruoka, Japan. For Reiko Kudo, a long battle of fighting cancer with real food taught her the undeniable link between food and health.

It's her mission to enable busy travelers to easily enjoy the benefits of real food. Japan and American both have work-centered societies, yet Japan acknowledges this busyness by incorporating a fast food culture that does not completely sacrifice quality. Instead of allowing lack of time to serve as an excuse for poor food, they have built a food infrastructure that supports it.

Much like how we allow many things to identify us, we also allow outside factors to determine and direct our usage of time. I do not minimalize the difficulties in combatting this, and I struggle with it frequently. The moment I think I've learned how to manage my time so that my calendar isn't completely full, something else (usually something I want to do) beckons for my attention. Not every opportunity is a calling or even something to pursue. "No," is a complete sentence. However, when our identity is seeking outward validation, it's difficult to discern where our time should be spent. This is because outward validation calls for us to have full schedules, for us to produce in order to have proof of our worth, and for our worth to be found in our doing. With all the doing, we miss what all the doing is for. A friend shared with me a mantra from her church that stuck with me. Being a food analogy, it doubly-resonated.

Make sushi, not fish stew.[3]

In Japan, there is a world-renowned sushi chef named Jiro Ono. Jiro, now in his 90s, has been making sushi for over sixty years. His life is an ode to sushi. His small, nondescript restaurant in Tokyo has served the world's dignitaries and is considered the finest sushi establishment in the world. He takes the best quality fish and honors its quality through simple, yet refined preparations. There is much depth in his simplicity. His sushi allows you to understand and appreciate the quality of the fish. However, if he took that fish and turned it into a fish stew, you would have to dig around to find the pieces of fish; they would be lost with everything around them. The finest piece of fish can't be appreciated when it's surrounded by so many other things, even if those things might also be the finest pieces of food as well. You might have bok choy and sweet onions, but by mixing them all together into a stew, you lose the simple depth of each. Jiro knew this, and so he chose to pursue sushi and to honor the quality of the ingredients through simplicity.

What is your fish stew? What is noble by intention but just a bit too muddied up to be honored or appreciated? The American work culture asks us to perform like sushi yet have the components of fish stew. They are not one and the same. By determining the non-negotiable pillars in your life (i.e. your "sushi"), you make time for those items first. Everything else gets slotted in. My sushi list is as follows:

1	Nourishing food
1	Family
1	Intentional friendships
1	Cultivating my faith
1	Passionate work
1	Natural movement
1	Quiet moments

Through this list, I desire to cultivate a life that honors my body, mind, and soul through nourishing food, quiet moments, natural movement, a faith that binds me, intentional family time and friendships to hold me, and passionate work that serves the world in which I live. I desire a life where I can savor a thick slice of fresh bread covered in peanut butter and banana with my morning coffee, a life where I would make time for a lunchtime walk and chat with a friend, and a life where I could end my day with yoga to thank it for the beauty of its natural movement. In this life, I would enjoy church service on Sundays without the preoccupied thoughts of everything that I wanted to check off my list before the week began again. I would be intentional with friendships and make that call to say, *I was thinking of you today. How are you?*

More times than I would care to admit, my sushi list looks more like the following:

1	Work
1	Obligations
1	Meetings
1	Frenzied movement
1	Busy mind

That list conjures up a much different kind of life, a life that looks nothing like the former list. I found myself backing out of social commitments due to my workload. When this trend didn't change, I simply stopped making social plans, knowing that there would be a high possibility that I would need to cancel. I ran from meeting to meeting, trying to quickly shift my mind from one project to the next. My mind was whirling, and still, I asked it to politely behave at the end of the day and allow me to sleep. I was irritable and moody. My good intentions ended up as fish stew. By not honoring the items on my list in and of themselves, I allowed them to blend together and morph so that they didn't resemble the life I desired. They became yet another to-do list. The thing is, we don't even see this happening if we don't anchor our actions in our identity.

When you determine your sushi list, you see what matters most to you. Make time for these things first. Like a healthy lifestyle, these are not one-hundred percent goals. Life happens. Sometimes you can't get a homemade meal, sometimes your day is more hectic than you'd like, and sometimes exercise doesn't happen. However, when day upon day looks quite different than what you'd like, it becomes time to take note and make a change. Your sushi list provides a guide for your days. You don't know how far you stray if you don't have a guidepost. With these non-negotiables listed out, you are better able to step back and analyze your days. Where are you prioritizing items that aren't even on your list? When do you have days where something simply needs to come off your list in order to get through it? The answers to these questions allow you to realistically approach your days. Since you are reading this, I'm assuming that nourishing food might be on your sushi list. Create and honor routines to make time for real food. Set yourself up for success by looking at your days and thinking about when you might need to have food on the go. Come at this from a very real place. Because nourishing food is important to me, I'll almost always have some type of food or snack in my bag. I don't like to be caught unaware and without food. For me, I know that it leads to snap decisions when I'm hungry. It's also OK to acknowledge that sometimes you need to stop somewhere for food. Or that you don't want to use the mind-space to figure out how and what you're doing to eat a day ahead of time and stopping somewhere is simply easier. The nutrition world can sometimes make us feel like failures if we don't eat something green at each meal. We're not. You're not. We're trying to do our best in a culture that makes it difficult to slow down, nourish, and reset. Set your pillars. Use them as guiding lights. They will alert you if you stray to a point where you're no longer comfortable with your compromises.

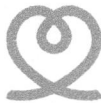

SUGGESTED PROJECT: WHAT'S ON YOUR SUSHI LIST?

Write out your desired sushi list, or your guiding pillars. Write out how you would like these to play out in your days and weeks. Then, write out what your current sushi list looks like. Are there overlaps, or are the two lists out of alignment? Take this information and analyze how you can honor your desires and anchor your days around your most important priorities.

Section III:
RECLAIMING OUR PLACE AT THE TABLE

We've explored who we are as eaters and the American food environment. We now need to turn our attention to how we use these insights to reclaim our place at the table—with knowledge, pleasure, and grace.

CHAPTER 9

THE NUTRITIONAL FORK IN THE ROAD

"We've gone from an environment of hardship and scarcity to one of abundance and ease. How can we make the most of this abundance without letting it ruin our health?"[1]

DAN BUETTNER

American history is rife with examples of perseverance and determination. As we've emerged from challenges in our more recent history, we've clung to the abundance with which we identify. This national identity and how it manifests at the table—the restaurant and home table alike—requires that we have more diligence and knowledge about the food on our tables. I wish it weren't so. Every time I've returned to America after living abroad, I've grappled with the dichotomy of our food. I celebrate the diversity and availability of ingredients from all over the world. *Gochujang* from Korea? No problem. *Katsuobushi* from Japan? We've got that too. Items that were mostly unheard of and unavailable in the tiny Italian town in which I lived are readily available in American grocery stores. Despite the joy of finding such a cornucopia of international foods in the American market, I found myself missing the simplicity of easily finding high-quality ingredients in Italian markets. Food was not expensive, farmer's markets were a regular occurrence and easily accessible, and items in the grocery stores were less adulterated. Most fruits and vegetables were seasonal and had the flavor that only an in-season food can bring. It made cooking a joy; I didn't have to do much to showcase the natural flavor that was already there. As long as I didn't need international ingredients, shopping and cooking were easy. However, being American, I was accustomed to living down the street from a Vietnamese shopping and restaurant center that had been featured by the likes of Anthony Bourdain. Little Korea was ten minutes in the other direction. Japanese cuisine? I could either buy the ingredients or go to any of the many Japanese restaurants that surrounded my home. Laotian? Also, not a problem. I had the world's food at my fingertips.

Living in Italy gave me a deep appreciation of the simplicity of cooking, the beauty of regional specialties, and the joy of lingering around a dinner table. It also imparted in me an unexpected appreciation for my home country. We don't have a flavor that defines us. Instead, we're a beautiful collection in America, and that results in many flavors that define us. I became grateful for my Italian-American family and the plethora of foods that I was exposed to from a young age in America. Our strength lies in our diversity. The question remains: will we harness this strength to find our place at the table?

JAMES AND THE GIANT PEACH

I remember when I went to the farmer's market soon after I moved to Italy and I found large, beautiful golden peaches. On a tight student's budget, I decided I'd splurge on these peaches. I told the grower that I'd take six of them, expecting to fully use my five-euro bill. Instead, I was shocked to hear my total was ninety-eight cents. Ninety-eight cents! I could spend less than a euro for juicy peaches that would last an entire week. I ate them as a snack, cooked them into my morning oatmeal, and made a dessert of peaches over sweetened sticky rice. All of this for so little.

I don't know of any farmer's market in America where I could find peaches for so little. Fair prices for labor are a large factor in this equation, and it is a topic that I will not do injustice to in so little space. My point here is that farmer's markets prices were much lower than what I had experienced in America. It made shopping at farmer's markets possible. This, in turn, meant that I could experience the weekly joy of speaking with producers, getting a free bundle of *pepperoncini* thrown in with my produce, and learning how to use what I was purchasing from the people behind the stand. These small exchanges brought immeasurable joy to my days and added human interactions to the process of cooking.

If food familiarity begets taste preferences, then we need to become less familiar with what is cheap and fast and more acquainted with what is nourishing and good. As our local eateries become replaced with large-scale chain restaurants, where the food is shipped in from far-away distribution centers, our plates become less meaningful and our palates are standardized. These chain restaurants, flourishing in a land of immigrants who came with the hopes of creating better lives, tap into a deeply-seated American value with their inexpensive large servings of food: abundance and access.[2] It hits upon the same cultural value that allowed large-scale supermarkets to flourish. American perseverance and determination will continue to drive our values and what we find on the table. Neglecting this fact ignores the very fabric of what it means to be American.

However, this value of more for less has led to the current state of poor health. The American love for abundance has fed a food industry that constantly creates new food products for needs we didn't know we had, and new nutritional guidance spawns the creation of nutritionally-changed processed foods. Yet, the industry is happy to find the solution to our ill-health in our lack of movement. American public service announcements will encourage kids to move more right before advertising a sugar-laden processed food. This disconnect is rampant in American culture, found in the dichotomy of abundance and personal responsibility, of good and bad food; yet, all of these do not account for why we eat in the first place.[3]

I've argued for the role of the individual in changing a nation plagued by ill-health, one meal at a time. There is no doubt that the system needs to be fixed to provide affordable access to healthy food, but I am arguing for a conscious eater in a damaged food system as well as a functional one. The food system will always be financially incentivized to take shortcuts when it comes to processed food.[4] An unaware consumer will let this happen again and again. Additionally, the food system has no incentive to change if the tastes and demands of the consumers do not force it. Until our eating habits change, the food system will continue to meet our sugared and salted demands.[5] Telling an individual to eat less without mentioning food quality is empty advice. You are telling the person to ignore their bio-computer that is programmed for real nutrition. The push for individual informed choice also forgets the other half of the eating equation: eating is a social activity that is shaped by our surroundings. This mentality leaves out the pleasures of the table.

Claude Fischler, a French social scientist, researched how different cultures value their experiences at the table. His comparative international data showed that quality produce, tradition, and the experiences of social eating were important to the French, Italians, and Swiss. Americans and the British, on the other hand, were more concerned with free and responsible individual choice, even expressing anxiety over this point. Americans showed a stronger inclination toward individual free choice than any of the six countries Fischler studied.[6] It's important to understand country and cultural differences when analyzing how to positively impact how people feed themselves. We need to understand how we can utilize traditional wisdom to re-engage our guttural sense of how to eat and live in an individualized, American context. Otherwise, we can continue to wait for nutritional science to enlighten us and show us what should be on our table—and eventually how we should come to it. Buettner points out the fallacy of the current tactic of telling people to diet and exercise in that it exhausts the willpower muscle through the monotony of routine. He details how this goes "against human nature and our evolutionary design. The human psyche craves the new and the novel."[7] We try to grab onto the latest superfood as our newest guardian of health without realizing that even that trend will not be novel for long. Studies have not found a single food in particular that is linked to longevity. People in the Blue Zones consume many fruits and vegetables of all colors, not only providing a wide range of nutrients, but also providing the variety that humans crave.[8]

We ask nutritional science to provide this level of narrow analysis when it comes to how we should eat. If we seek health and the enjoyment that comes from it then we need to broaden the lens to look at food as a whole, not as a sum of its parts. Nutritional findings should be conveyed in ways that incorporate both the quality of food as an important factor, as well as the cultural context.[9] For example, we are currently consuming large quantities of soy products as they have been endorsed by nutrition experts for their health properties. Understanding soy consumption in a cultural context would have told us that soy is traditionally fermented in Japan before consumption. Nutritionism merely told us that soy could be healthy, spawning the availability of unfermented soy products in America. When health advice is not contextualized, we miss the point, again and again. Health experts learned about the Okinawan saying, *hara hachi bu*, and started to promote its use and the lesson it contains. While a valid lesson, it ignores the fact that a toxic and processed food system is not one that you should be consuming until you are eighty percent full. In the American context, we need to first re-engage our understanding of what real food is before we begin to practice *hara hachi bu*. A cautious and humble approach to nutrition would have balanced our inclination toward the new and novel. It would have told us to be suspicious of margarine and not dictate that our fat consumption not exceed thirty percent of our total calories. It would have shown us that people in the Mediterranean eat upwards of forty percent of their calories in fat.[10] It would have told us that there is wisdom and health in diets that have supported our existence for millenniums. It would have empowered us to trust our own abilities to feed ourselves before we strayed so far away.

As humans who crave variety, we have plenty on American land. We are now at a crossroads where we need to figure out what to do with it, and how to use our abundance to positively enrich our health and lives instead of diminishing it. We have the world's food at our fingertips. Unfortunately, we also have a food system and culture that lack the world's wisdom on how to form and maintain healthy relationships with food. We're still a young nation, and I was reminded of that as I traveled around the world. Throughout my interviews, people would tell me that their countries had made many mistakes and learned from them. They were reticent to adopt new fads or changes to their food supply. Like most things, this has its positives as well as drawbacks. I've come to appreciate America's willingness to break down barriers and approach challenges with wonder and ingenuity. We don't willingly say "No" to things until we've tried, and even then, we are apt to continue to experiment and improvise. As Fischler's research pointed out, Americans like individual free choice.[11] We've revolutionized our food system, and abundant food and access has come from that. We now need to refine and correct the errors that have emerged. This is a normal part of the process and it speaks to our collective identity as Americans. We were never meant to be passive consumers of a system, but instead a people who constantly analyze, evaluate, and fight for the better. We're called to pay attention, and our health and nutrition is no different. Most changes in America have started at the individual level before they ever touched our national identity. Our relationship with food is currently at that fork in the road.

Chapter 10

COME TO THE TABLE

"Slowness is a metaphor for understanding and enjoyment, of being able to know who you are and what you taste."[1]

Carlo Petrini

At this table, in this space, you are welcome here. You are welcome to bring your story, your challenges, and your triumphs. You are welcome to work through them. You are welcome to rewrite your story. When we see how food systems can support or undermine healthy decisions, we realize how little we understood about the food on our tables. Travel serves to reframe how we view food and the food choices presented to us. It has for me, and it's my hope that these small glimpses into the world tables, along with a better understanding of nutrition history in America, have helped to recalibrate your thoughts on food and even just a sliver of all that is contained within it.

Numerous leaders and entrepreneurs report that their secret to success lies in their ability to reframe failures as learning opportunities. Where perceived failures are enough to halt even the most determined, others see them as opportunities, a lens through which to better understand their objectives, their mission, and what they believe in. This cycle is iterative and happens over and over, each time providing a chance to refocus and refine. The path of an intuitive eater is no different. There will be challenges and struggles that come with your decision to reclaim your relationship with food. Celebrate them. For they, too, allow you to understand how you relate to the table. If we change our focus from an analysis of nutrient content to an openness toward the enjoyment of the flavors of real food, then we might find that we are able to tap into the importance of the simplicity of coming to the table. Both the French and the Italians structure their days around mealtimes. They honor it, the food, and the people they share it with. After traveling, Italians will often ask you, "So, did you eat well?" This question embodies the Italian spirit around the role of food. To eat well is to live well. If you ate well while traveling, then the assumption follows that you were well taken care of.

Our binary views of food, the body, and pleasure have roots in the cultural norms of the Middle Ages. Pleasure was a slippery slope of which one should be weary. Eating, a necessary activity, was made less pleasurable through medieval cooking techniques targeting the reduction of pleasure. It was thought that food should be consumed for health only, not for the enjoyment of it, should it lead one down a path of excess.[2] We continue to see the pervasiveness of this mentality in nutritionism. We are told to eat soy because it is good for us, even though our culture has no prior relationship with soy. We are pushed to eat more nuts because of the omega-3 fats they contain.[3] We need to break with this reductive and antiquated thinking. Instead of seeking omega-3s, I would encourage us to eat the almond—in a pesto, as a snack, on a salad, however you wish—but always with enjoyment and a conscious understanding that the food you are eating serves you both nutritionally and spiritually. This is where knowledge meets pleasure and the metabolism of passion takes over.

We need to learn to be kind to ourselves. The words we use hold power. The more we recognize that being kind can take the shape of pizza as much as it can also be a spinach and quinoa salad, the more we release the pressure of the binge and restrict spectrum. We allow ourselves to make peace with the table and, in turn, with ourselves. The following chart details many of the words and phrases we use, consciously and subconsciously. I've outlined where these fall on the binge/restrict spectrum and how we can reframe them to build a language of acceptance and love—a language that supports our own individual metabolisms of passion. You'll note that some of these fall on both ends of the spectrum as we binge one day with the anticipation of restricting the next.

	BINGE/ RESTRICT	WHAT WE ARE SAYING TO OURSELVES	REFRAMED WORD/ PHRASE
Cheat Day/ Cheating/ Cheat Meal	Binge	I feel restricted in my day-to-day food choices and am tired of exerting control over my food. I want to have a meal/day where I am not fighting to convince myself to eat healthy over what I truly want to eat.	I choose to have a pleasurable meal that serves my human desire for variety. Every food day does not need to look the same. Our ability to eat a variety of foods should be celebrated!
Guilty Pleasure	Binge	This is a bad food and I shouldn't allow myself to indulge.	This is food I take great pleasure in. It is neither good nor bad. I've been nourishing my body in many ways and will enjoy this food.

	BINGE/ RESTRICT	WHAT WE ARE SAYING TO OURSELVES	REFRAMED WORD/ PHRASE
I'm on a diet	Restrict	I am seeking to change something in my life and am exerting control over my food in an attempt to attain what I feel is lacking.	95% of diets fail because they do not serve the humans who are on them. Instead of going on another diet, I will learn to listen to my bodily hunger/satiety clues to better understand the language of my body and what it requires.
I'm holding a food funeral/ I'm working up to when I'll start the diet	Binge and Restrict	Healthy food is not delicious and cannot hold pleasure. I can only gain pleasure from foods that I crave and delight in. There is no room for balance, so I will over-in-dulge with foods I love and deem "unhealthy" with the goal of going on a diet soon and restricting these foods from my life.	I'm willing to learn what foods serve my body and what I also enjoy. I can allow my body to teach me what it needs by eating nutritious foods and understanding that intuitive eating does not qualify foods as good or bad, nor does it eliminate whole food groups.

	BINGE/ RESTRICT	WHAT WE ARE SAYING TO OURSELVES	REFRAMED WORD/ PHRASE
I already ate X and ruined it today so no use start-ing tomorrow.	Binge	I ate horribly and messed up my diet. It makes no difference if I eat well today be-cause I messed up so badly already.	Ruined what? I had a pleasurable meal. Great! Now I will thank my body for allowing a plethora of eating experiences and will give it some love back by caring for it. Love first, always. I care for my body not out of guilt, restriction, or punishment.
I shouldn't eat that.	Restrict	This is a bad food and will cause me to gain weight. I shouldn't give in to my human desire to crave certain foods.	I understand that there are no restrictions and I am in-tune with my body to understand what I desire to eat or not eat. I don't choose to restrict foods from a place of deprivation and denial.

This reframing of everyday expressions is where the metabolism of passion informs our food choices and how we experience them. As we've explored, much of our food environment is out of our control. Despite this, I believe we should be aware of the outside pressures around us, and how these influence our day to day thoughts and action. This is why we begin with knowledge—the knowledge of a broken food system and a diet culture that bombards us daily with messages of inadequacy and willpower—to strengthen our understanding of the world in which we live. We build an ability to see through the nonsense and, in turn, the nonsense becomes less able to penetrate our psyche and influence how we view ourselves and how we come to the table. This clears the way for us to do the work of pleasure. I do not take this work lightly. To approach the table with pleasure and appreciation in a culture that made the pleasures of the table akin to gluttony is no easy feat. It feels as though we're turning our back on everything we know and hold true. This is because, for many of us, we were never taught that the pleasures of the table are rightfully ours. More importantly, we were never given permission—or, gave ourselves permission—to pursue them with gusto and to actually seek them out. Furthermore, the dichotomies of being a woman have plagued how we come to the table: informed but delightfully unaware; interested but not too much; open but also reserved. Much of our language around the table stems from this pressure to be everything and all, and never too much.

I want to eat that cake, but I shouldn't.
Chocolate, fudgy cookies are my guilty pleasure.
Pizza is my cheat meal.

Listen to the underlying feelings in these phrases.

I want to eat that cake, but I shouldn't. (I'm tired of fighting my desires.)
Chocolate, fudgy cookies are my guilty pleasure. (Because if I were sensible and in control of my life I wouldn't crave them.)
Pizza is my cheat meal. (I really enjoy pizza.)

Release it. All of it. Enjoying food doesn't make you weak or any less than. The pleasures of the table are for everyone, as is a deep understanding of what foods serve our bodies at various times. Adam Gopnik summarizes this balance in *The Table Comes First*: "Life is a whole—that we can live fully and that we ought to, with our pleasures as much as with our principles."[4] *Pleasure and knowledge*. It's how to build an understanding of our own unique metabolism of passion and what it means to each of us. It's how we remind ourselves to be gentle with the journey. It's how we make sense of our country's nutritional confusion and move forward with amusement and curiosity. The table is not absent from the daily challenges and noise. Making peace with it means that you can be in the midst of these things and still seek nourishment and pleasure at the table. Eating for nourishment is as important as eating for enjoyment, and you can bring a calm knowing to the center of the chaos.

We eat three times a day. In a year's time, this amounts to over one thousand opportunities to choose health and enjoyment.[5] An intuitive eater understands the balance implicit in this number. This allows for celebratory meals without guilt or anxiety when your foundation is an understanding of real food and the joy it can bring. We need to practice this before we lose our instinctual knowledge of how to eat and what it means. Food pleasure need not be at odds with health. In fact, health demands the company of pleasure. Healthy food cultures have long understood this beautiful balance. It's long-overdue for this message to land in America. Food as a daily source of pleasure holds the power to nourish us, body and soul, if we just allow it to do so. Our misguided culture may have blurred the lines of what a healthy relationship with food looks like, but it is time we pick up our forks, empowered with the knowledge of how to feed ourselves. Until then, you can find me at the table eating joyfully. I invite you to join me there, so I can ask you: Did you eat well?

ACKNOWLEDGEMENTS

To my mom and dad, thank you for being my biggest cheerleaders. You've always believed in me and even encouraged me to pick up my life and move to Italy to pursue my passion. You told me to take a risk even when I was reticent. You never hesitate to tell anyone within earshot that your daughter got her master's degree in Italy. Thank you for working so hard to give me the opportunities I've been blessed to experience. Thank you for sharing in the joys and pains alike.

Genevieve Crum, I don't have the words to thank you for your tireless editing. You give such structure and clarity to my thoughts and words. This book would not exist without you and our countless bike rides and coffee working sessions in Italy discussing the American food system, nutrition, and health. Thank you for caring so deeply about these issues that you'd wax poetic about them hour upon hour, each time helping me clarify my thoughts on how to incorporate our studies and experiences back at the American table. All of these conversations gave birth to this book, one cappuccino at a time (but never after breakfast).

Tien Bui, your keen eye and your humor brought a needed lightness to the editing process. You comically guided me to get rid of excess words and tighten up my writing. My words no longer have the feeling of eating a kebab after an indulgent Italian dinner, as you so wittily put it. Thank you for walking through this with me.

Thank you to the Institute for Integrative Nutrition and the University of Gastronomic Sciences for providing the intellectual paths for me to pursue my deep love affair with all things food. Thank you to Gabriella Morini, Simone Cinotto, and Stanley Ulijaszek, among so many others, who shaped my master's experience and the formation of my thoughts on food, health, relationships, and the world. You opened up Italy and the food systems of the world to me and were instrumental in a fourteen-month period that will continue to shape the way I view how we come to the table.

Meg Tucker, thank you for your copyediting and attention to detail. To the guys behind Sandcastle, Foster and Kevin, I can't thank you enough for the book cover design and the interior layout. You had so much patience as we worked through each iteration and you brought my vision to life.

Thank you to the countless others over the years who have listened and nodded their heads as I spoke endlessly about the table, how we come to it, and the role of pleasure in solidifying strong relationships with food. This book would never exist without your willingness to listen, debate, and banter, all of which made me think and refine my thoughts about how we come to the table in America.

INDEX

ENDNOTES

INTRODUCTION: FOOD PLEASURE MATTERS

1   Young, Molly. "Lies We Tell Ourselves About Avocado Toast." Bon Appetit, 14 Mar. 2017, www.bonappetit.com/story/lies-about-avocado-toast.

2   Scrinis, Gyorgy. Nutritionism: The Science and Politics of Dietary Advice. New York: Columbia University Press, 2015, 234.

3   Nicola Perullo, 2016, 12 Perullo, Nicola, and Massimo Montanari. Taste as Experience: The Philosophy and Aesthetics of Food. New York: Columbia University Press, 2016, 12.

4   Simpson, Stephen J., and David Raubenheimer. "Perspective: Tricks of the Trade." Nature News. April 16, 2014. Accessed September 2017. http://www.nature.com/nature/journal/v508/n7496_supp/full/508S66a.html

5   Petrini, Carlo. Slow Food: The Case for Taste. New York: Columbia University Press, 2001, 20-21, 70.

6   "Passion." Merriam-Webster, Sept. 2017, www.merriam-webster.com/dictionary/passion.

7   "Pleasure." Merriam-Webster, Sept. 2017, www.merriam-webster.com/dictionary/pleasure.

8   "Pleasure." Oxford Dictionaries, Sept. 2017, en.oxforddictionaries.com/definition/pleasure.

9   "Metabolism." Dictionary.com, Sept. 2017, www.dictionary.com/browse/metabolism.

10 David, Marc. "The Metabolic Power of Pleasure." The Institute for the Psychology of Eating, 2014, psychologyofeating.com/metabolic-power-pleasure/.

11 Tandoh, Ruby. "The Unhealthy Truth Behind 'Wellness' and 'Clean Eating'." Vice, 13 May 2016, www.vice.com/en_us/article/jm5nvp/ruby-tandoh-eat-clean-wellness.

12 Scrinis, Gyorgy. Nutritionism: The Science and Politics of Dietary Advice. New York: Columbia University Press, 2015, 233.

CHAPTER 1: UNDERSTANDING OUR FOOD IDENTITIES

1   Wilson, Bee, and Annabel Lee. First Bite: How We Learn to Eat. Basic Books, 2016.

2   Buettner, Dan. The Blue Zones Solution: Eating and Living like the World's Healthiest People. Washington, DC: National Geographic Partners, 2015.

3   Birch, Leann L., and Allison E. Doub. "Learning to Eat: Birth to Age 2 Y." American Journal of Clinical Nutrition 99, no. 3 (2014). doi:10.3945/ajcn.113.069047, 725S.

4   Birch, Leann L., and Allison E. Doub. "Learning to Eat: Birth to Age 2 Y." American Journal of Clinical Nutrition 99, no. 3 (2014). doi:10.3945/ajcn.113.069047.

5   Petrini, Carlo. Slow Food: The Case for Taste. New York: Columbia University Press, 2001, 74.

6   Wilson, Bee, and Annabel Lee. First Bite: How We Learn to Eat. Basic Books, 2016.

CHAPTER 2: ON KALE AND QUINOA

1   "Obesity Update 2017." Obesity Update - OECD, Sept. 2017, www.oecd. org/health/obesity-update.htm.

2   "If You're Too Busy For These 5 Things: Your Life Is More Off-Course Than You Think." Thrive Global, 18 Sept. 2017, journal.thriveglobal. com/if-youre-too-busy-for-these-5-things-your-life-is-more-off-course-than-you-think-c2822830a38e.

CHAPTER 3: THERE'S A HOLE IN MY BUCKET

1   Osho. The Book of Wisdom: The Heart of Tibetan Buddhism. OSHO International, 2014.

2   "There's a Hole in My Bucket." Wikipedia, 31 Mar. 2018, en.wikipedia. org/wiki/There's_a_Hole_in_My_Bucket.

3   Brillat-Savarin, Jean Anthelme., and M.F.K Fischer. M.K.F. Fischer's Translation of the Physiology of Taste: or Meditations on Transcendental Gastronomy. Knopf, 1971.

4   Albala, Ken. "Food: A Cultural Culinary History." Audible.com, The Great Courses, 8 July 2013, www.audible.com/pd/History/Food-A-Cultural-Culinary-History-Audiobook/B00D8EMBVQ.

CHAPTER 4: CAN WE TALK ABOUT THE CHOCOLATE CAKE?

1   "Jens Stoltenberg Quotes." BrainyQuote.com. Xplore Inc, 2018. 31 March 2018. https://www.brainyquote.com/quotes/jens_stoltenberg_640351.

2   Buettner, Dan. The Blue Zones: Lessons for Living Longer from the People Who've Lived the Longest. Washington, D.C.: National Geographic Society, 2008.

CHAPTER 5: THE FIGHT FOR THE AMERICAN BREAKFAST TABLE

1   "Shojin Ryori Project." Aug. 2017, Tsuruoka , Japan.

2   N. Campbell-McBride, M.D. Gut and Psychology Syndrome. Journal of Orthomolecular Medicine Vol. 23, No. 2, 2008. https://pdfs.semanticscholar.org/72c4/0e26819994eaeff1e05e8e97bbba02a943fe.pdf#page=34

3   Furrow, Dwight. American Foodie: Taste, Art, and the Cultural Revolution. Lanham: Rowman & Littlefield, 2016, 11.

4   Scrinis, Gyorgy. Nutritionism: The Science and Politics of Dietary Advice. New York: Columbia University Press, 2015.

5   Bentley, Amy, and Hi'ilei Hobart. "Food in Recent U.S. History." In Food in Time and Place: The American Historical Association Companion to Food History, by Paul H. Freedman, Joyce E. Chaplin, and Ken Albala. Oakland, CA: University of California Press, 2014, 166.

6   Levenstein, Harvey A. Paradox of Plenty: A Social History of Eating in Modern America. Berkeley, CA: University of California Press, 1993

7   Scrinis, Gyorgy. Nutritionism: The Science and Politics of Dietary Advice. New York: Columbia University Press, 2015, 46.

8   Buettner, Dan. The Blue Zones Solution: Eating and Living like the World's Healthiest People. Washington, DC: National Geographic Partners, 2015.

9   Scrinis, Gyorgy. Nutritionism: The Science and Politics of Dietary Advice. New York: Columbia University Press, 2015, 59.

10 Bentley, Amy, and Hi'ilei Hobart. "Food in Recent U.S. History." In Food in Time and Place: The American Historical Association Companion to Food History, by Paul H. Freedman, Joyce E. Chaplin, and Ken Albala. Oakland, CA: University of California Press, 2014, 168.

11   Levenstein, Harvey A. Paradox of Plenty: A Social History of Eating in Modern America. Berkeley, CA: University of California Press, 1993, 6.

12   "Norman Borlaug - Biographical." Nobelprize.org, www.nobelprize.org/nobel_prizes/peace/laureates/1970/borlaug-bio.html.

13   Bentley, Amy, and Hi'ilei Hobart. "Food in Recent U.S. History." In Food in Time and Place: The American Historical Association Companion to Food History, by Paul H. Freedman, Joyce E. Chaplin, and Ken Albala. Oakland, CA: University of California Press, 2014, 169.

14   Bentley, Amy, and Hi'ilei Hobart. "Food in Recent U.S. History." In Food in Time and Place: The American Historical Association Companion to Food History, by Paul H. Freedman, Joyce E. Chaplin, and Ken Albala. Oakland, CA: University of California Press, 2014,, 169-170.

15   Bentley, Amy, and Hi'ilei Hobart. "Food in Recent U.S. History." In Food in Time and Place: The American Historical Association Companion to Food History, by Paul H. Freedman, Joyce E. Chaplin, and Ken Albala. Oakland, CA: University of California Press, 2014, 170-172.

16   Furrow, Dwight. American Foodie: Taste, Art, and the Cultural Revolution. Lanham: Rowman & Littlefield, 2016, 7.

17   Scrinis, Gyorgy. Nutritionism: The Science and Politics of Dietary Advice. New York: Columbia University Press, 2015.

18   Scrinis, Gyorgy. Nutritionism: The Science and Politics of Dietary Advice. New York: Columbia University Press, 2015.

19   Ulijaszek, Stanley, Neil Mann, and Sarah Elton. "Evolving Human Nutrition." 2012. doi:10.1017/cbo9781139046794.

20   Scrinis, Gyorgy. Nutritionism: The Science and Politics of Dietary Advice. New York: Columbia University Press, 2015, 82.

21   Scrinis, Gyorgy. Nutritionism: The Science and Politics of Dietary Advice. New York: Columbia University Press, 2015, 7, 86-87.

22   Bentley, Amy, and Hi'ilei Hobart. "Food in Recent U.S. History." In Food in Time and Place: The American Historical Association Companion to Food History, by Paul H. Freedman, Joyce E. Chaplin, and Ken Albala. Oakland, CA: University of California Press, 2014, 173.

23   Scrinis, Gyorgy. Nutritionism: The Science and Politics of Dietary Advice. New York: Columbia University Press, 2015, 46, 158.

24 Scrinis, Gyorgy. Nutritionism: The Science and Politics of Dietary Advice. New York: Columbia University Press, 2015, 158.

25 Scrinis, Gyorgy. Nutritionism: The Science and Politics of Dietary Advice. New York: Columbia University Press, 2015, 12.

26 Scrinis, Gyorgy. Nutritionism: The Science and Politics of Dietary Advice. New York: Columbia University Press, 2015, 174.

27 Scrinis, Gyorgy. Nutritionism: The Science and Politics of Dietary Advice. New York: Columbia University Press, 2015, 211.

28 Bentley, Amy, and Hi'ilei Hobart. "Food in Recent U.S. History." In Food in Time and Place: The American Historical Association Companion to Food History, by Paul H. Freedman, Joyce E. Chaplin, and Ken Albala. Oakland, CA: University of California Press, 2014, 179, 180, 182.

29 Miller, Bryan. "Prescriptions for Dining Out: 2 Health Experts Face Menus." The New York Times, 16 Apr. 1986, www.nytimes.com/1986/04/16/garden/prescriptions-for-dining-out-2-health-experts-face-menus.html.

30 Scrinis, Gyorgy. Nutritionism: The Science and Politics of Dietary Advice. New York: Columbia University Press, 2015, 2.

31 Scrinis, Gyorgy. Nutritionism: The Science and Politics of Dietary Advice. New York: Columbia University Press, 2015, 5.

32 "Office of Dietary Supplements - Vitamin A." NIH Office of Dietary Supplements, U.S. Department of Health and Human Services, ods.od.nih.gov/factsheets/VitaminA-HealthProfessional/.

33 Office of Dietary Supplements - Vitamin A." NIH Office of Dietary Supplements, U.S. Department of Health and Human Services, ods.od.nih.gov/factsheets/VitaminA-HealthProfessional/.

34 Scrinis, Gyorgy. Nutritionism: The Science and Politics of Dietary Advice. New York: Columbia University Press, 2015, 4-6.

35 Scrinis, Gyorgy. Nutritionism: The Science and Politics of Dietary Advice. New York: Columbia University Press, 2015, 7.

36 "TIME Magazine Cover: Cholesterol - Mar. 26, 1984." Time, Time Inc., content.time.com/time/covers/0,16641,19840326,00.html.

37 Time. "Fat Is Good for You." Time, Time, time.com/2863227/ending-the-war-on-fat/.

38 Scrinis, Gyorgy. Nutritionism: The Science and Politics of Dietary Advice. New York: Columbia University Press, 2015, 4.

39   Scrinis, Gyorgy. Nutritionism: The Science and Politics of Dietary Advice. New York: Columbia University Press, 2015, 13.

40   Scrinis, Gyorgy. Nutritionism: The Science and Politics of Dietary Advice. New York: Columbia University Press, 2015, 28, 29, 178.

41   Furrow, Dwight. American Foodie: Taste, Art, and the Cultural Revolution. Lanham: Rowman & Littlefield, 2016, 157.

42   Kearney, John. "Food Consumption Trends and Drivers." Philosophical Transactions of the Royal Society B: Biological Sciences, vol. 365, no. 1554, 2010, pp. 2793–2807., doi:10.1098/rstb.2010.0149.

43   Popkin, Barry M. "The Nutrition Transition in the Developing World." Development Policy Review, vol. 21, no. 5-6, 2003, pp. 581–597., doi:10.1111/j.1467-8659.2003.00225.x.

44   Lenoir, Magalie, et al. "Intense Sweetness Surpasses Cocaine Reward." PLoS ONE, vol. 2, no. 8, 2007, doi:10.1371/journal.pone.0000698.

45   Popkin, Barry M. "The Nutrition Transition in the Developing World." Development Policy Review, vol. 21, no. 5-6, 2003, pp. 581–597., doi:10.1111/j.1467-8659.2003.00225.x.

46   Scrinis, Gyorgy. Nutritionism: The Science and Politics of Dietary Advice. New York: Columbia University Press, 2015, 30, 113, 116, 117.

CHAPTER 6: THE INGREDIENTS OF HEALTHY FOOD CULTURES

1   Scrinis, Gyorgy. Nutritionism: The Science and Politics of Dietary Advice. New York: Columbia University Press, 2015, 216.

2   "Morbidity." Merriam-Webster, www.merriam-webster.com/dictionary/morbidity.

3   "The Original 'Blue Zones.'" Blue Zones, bluezones.com/live-longer-better/original-blue-zones/#section-1.

4   Buettner, Dan. The Blue Zones Solution: Eating and Living like the World's Healthiest People. Washington, DC: National Geographic Partners, 2015.

5   Buettner, Dan. The Blue Zones Solution: Eating and Living like the World's Healthiest People. Washington, DC: National Geographic Partners, 2015.

6   Buettner, Dan. The Blue Zones Solution: Eating and Living like the World's Healthiest People. Washington, DC: National Geographic Partners, 2015.

7   "The Original 'Blue Zones.'" Blue Zones, bluezones.com/
     live-longer-better/original-blue-zones/#section-1.

8   Scrinis, Gyorgy. Nutritionism: The Science and Politics of Dietary
     Advice. New York: Columbia University Press, 2015, 227.

9   Scrinis, Gyorgy. Nutritionism: The Science and Politics of Dietary
     Advice. New York: Columbia University Press, 2015, 227.

10   Buettner, Dan. The Blue Zones Solution: Eating and Living like the
     World's Healthiest People. Washington, DC: National Geographic
     Partners, 2015.

11   Frank, John. "Origins of the Obesity Pandemic Can Be
     Analysed." Nature News, 13 Apr. 2016, www.nature.com/news/
     origins-of-the-obesity-pandemic-can-be-analysed-1.19744.

12   Miller, Daphne, and Allison Sarubin-Fragakis. The Jungle Effect:
     A Doctor Discovers the Healthiest Diets from around the World--
     Why They Work and How to Bring Them Home. New York: Collins,
     2008, 42.

13   Miller, Daphne, and Allison Sarubin-Fragakis. The Jungle Effect:
     A Doctor Discovers the Healthiest Diets from around the World--
     Why They Work and How to Bring Them Home. New York: Collins,
     2008, 24.

14   "Convivial." Merriam-Webster, www.merriam-webster.com/
     dictionary/convivial.

15   "The Original 'Blue Zones.'" Blue Zones, bluezones.com/
     live-longer-better/original-blue-zones/#section-1.

16   Buettner, Dan. The Blue Zones: Lessons for Living Longer from
     the People Who've Lived the Longest. Washington, D.C.: National
     Geographic Society, 2008.

17   Buettner, Dan. The Blue Zones Solution: Eating and Living like the
     World's Healthiest People. Washington, DC: National Geographic
     Partners, 2015.

18   Buettner, Dan. The Blue Zones Solution: Eating and Living like the
     World's Healthiest People. Washington, DC: National Geographic
     Partners, 2015.

19   Buettner, Dan. The Blue Zones Solution: Eating and Living like the
     World's Healthiest People. Washington, DC: National Geographic
     Partners, 2015.

20   Miller, Daphne, and Allison Sarubin-Fragakis. The Jungle Effect: A
     Doctor Discovers the Healthiest Diets from around the World-- Why

They Work and How to Bring Them Home. New York: Collins, 2008, 27.

21   Furrow, Dwight. American Foodie: Taste, Art, and the Cultural Revolution. Lanham: Rowman & Littlefield, 2016, 64.

22   Scrinis, Gyorgy. Nutritionism: The Science and Politics of Dietary Advice. New York: Columbia University Press, 2015, 229-230.

23   Buettner, Dan. The Blue Zones Solution: Eating and Living like the World's Healthiest People. Washington, DC: National Geographic Partners, 2015.

24   Scrinis, Gyorgy. Nutritionism: The Science and Politics of Dietary Advice. New York: Columbia University Press, 2015, 237.

25   Buettner, Dan. The Blue Zones Solution: Eating and Living like the World's Healthiest People. Washington, DC: National Geographic Partners, 2015.

26   Miller, Daphne, and Allison Sarubin-Fragakis. The Jungle Effect: A Doctor Discovers the Healthiest Diets from around the World-- Why They Work and How to Bring Them Home. New York: Collins, 2008, 53.

27   Miller, Daphne, and Allison Sarubin-Fragakis. The Jungle Effect: A Doctor Discovers the Healthiest Diets from around the World-- Why They Work and How to Bring Them Home. New York: Collins, 2008, 56.

CHAPTER 8: SUSHI, NOT FISH STEW

1   Pieper, Josef, and Alexander Dru. Leisure, the Basis of Culture. Collins, 1965.

2   Safi, Omid. "Awakin.org." Awakin RSS, 20 June 2016, www.awakin. org/read/view.php?tid=2164.

3   Miller, Jason. South Bend City Church sermon January 25, 2018.

CHAPTER 9: THE NUTRITIONAL FORK IN THE ROAD

1   Buettner, Dan. The Blue Zones Solution: Eating and Living like the World's Healthiest People. Washington, DC: National Geographic Partners, 2015.

2   Filipovic, Jill. "The Way America Eats Is Killing Us. Something Has to Change." The Guardian. September 26, 2013. Accessed September

2017. https://www.theguardian.com/commentisfree/2013/sep/26/american-diet-report-card-unhealty.

3   Julier, Alice. "The Political Economy of Obesity." In Food and Culture: A Reader, by Carole Counihan and Penny Van Esterik. 2nd ed. New York: Routledge, 2008, 488-490.

4   Scrinis, Gyorgy. Nutritionism: The Science and Politics of Dietary Advice. New York: Columbia University Press, 2015, 13.

5   Mead, Margaret. "The Problem of Changing Food Habits." In Food and Culture: A Reader, by Carole Counihan and Penny Van Esterik. 2nd ed. New York: Routledge, 2008, 22, 25.

6   Fischler, Claude. "The Nutritional Cacophony May Be Detrimental to Your Health." Progress in Nutrition, November 2011.

7   Buettner, Dan. The Blue Zones Solution: Eating and Living like the World's Healthiest People. Washington, DC: National Geographic Partners, 2015

8   Buettner, Dan. The Blue Zones Solution: Eating and Living like the World's Healthiest People. Washington, DC: National Geographic Partners, 2015.

9   Scrinis, Gyorgy. Nutritionism: The Science and Politics of Dietary Advice. New York: Columbia University Press, 2015, 236.

10   Scrinis, Gyorgy. Nutritionism: The Science and Politics of Dietary Advice. New York: Columbia University Press, 2015, 227, 231, 244.

11   Fischler, Claude. "The Nutritional Cacophony May Be Detrimental to Your Health." Progress in Nutrition, November 2011.

CHAPTER 10: COME TO THE TABLE

1   Furrow, Dwight. American Foodie: Taste, Art, and the Cultural Revolution. Lanham: Rowman & Littlefield, 2016.

2   Petrini, Carlo. Slow Food: The Case for Taste. New York: Columbia University Press, 2001, 21-24.

3   Scrinis, Gyorgy. Nutritionism: The Science and Politics of Dietary Advice. New York: Columbia University Press, 2015, 253.

4   Gopnik, Adam. The Table Comes First: Family, France, and the Meaning of Food. London: Quercus, 2012.

5   Buettner, Dan. The Blue Zones Solution: Eating and Living like the World's Healthiest People. Washington, DC: National Geographic Partners, 2015.

MEET THE AUTHOR

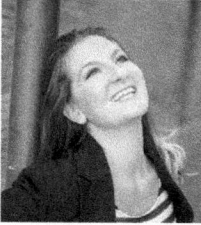

Tiffany Bassford is a Certified International Health Coach who left her ten-year corporate career to move to Italy to earn her Master of Gastronomy. She immersed herself in the study of global food cultures to learn first-hand about the role of pleasure at the table. She completed her thesis research in Japan and wrote her master's thesis on healthy food cultures and how to adapt those lessons to the American table.

Tiffany's approach to the table is one of grace, amusement, and curiosity. She believes that the table provides a meeting place for us to better understand who we are as eaters and how we show up in life. Her coaching practice pairs food knowledge with food pleasure to create meaningful relationships with food and yourself that endure.

For more information visit:
www.foodpassionproject.com

www.ingramcontent.com/pod-product-compliance
Lightning Source LLC
Chambersburg PA
CBHW060503280326
41933CB00014B/2842